New Technologies in Spine Surgery

Editors

NATHANIEL P. BROOKS
MICHAEL Y. WANG

NEUROSURGERY
CLINICS OF NORTH AMERICA

www.neurosurgery.theclinics.com

Consulting Editors
RUSSELL R. LONSER
DANIEL K. RESNICK

January 2020 • Volume 31 • Number 1

ELSEVIER

1600 John F. Kennedy Boulevard • Suite 1800 • Philadelphia, Pennsylvania, 19103-2899

http://www.theclinics.com

NEUROSURGERY CLINICS OF NORTH AMERICA Volume 31, Number 1
January 2020 ISSN 1042-3680, ISBN-13: 978-0-323-70933-0

Editor: Katerina Heidhausen
Developmental Editor: Laura Fisher

Neurosurgery Clinics of North America (ISSN 1042-3680) is published quarterly by Elsevier Inc., 360 Park Avenue South, New York, NY 10010-1710. Months of issue are January, April, July, and October. Business and Editorial Offices: 1600 John F. Kennedy Blvd., Suite 1800, Philadelphia, PA 19103-2899. Customer Service Office: 11830 Westline Industrial Drive, St. Louis, MO 63146. Periodicals postage paid at New York, NY, and additional mailing offices. Subscription prices are $434.00 per year (US individuals), $785.00 per year (US institutions), $470.00 per year (Canadian individuals), $974.00 per year (Canadian institutions), $534.00 per year (international individuals), $974.00 per year (international institutions), $100.00 per year (US students), $255.00 per year (international students), and $100.00 per year (Canadian students). International air speed delivery is included in all *Clinics* subscription prices. All prices are subject to change without notice. **POSTMASTER:** Send address changes to *Neurosurgery Clinics of North America*, Elsevier Periodicals Customer Service, 11830 Westline Industrial Drive, St. Louis, MO 63146. **Customer Service: 1-800-654-2452 (US and Canada). From outside the US and Canada, call: 1-314-453-7041. Fax: 1-314-453-5170. E-mail: JournalsCustomerService-usa@elsevier.com (for print support) and journalsonline-support-usa@elsevier.com (for online support).**

Reprints. For copies of 100 or more, of articles in this publication, please contact the Commercial Reprints Department, Elsevier Inc., 360 Park Avenue South, New York, NY 10010-1710. Tel. 212-633-3874; Fax: 212-633-3820; E-mail: reprints@elsevier.com.

Neurosurgery Clinics of North America is covered in *MEDLINE/PubMed (Index Medicus), EMBASE/Excerpta Medica, and Current Contents/Clinical Medicine (CC/CM).*

Contributors

CONSULTING EDITORS

RUSSELL R. LONSER, MD
Professor and Chair, Department of
Neurological Surgery, The Ohio State
University Wexner Medical Center, Columbus,
Ohio, USA

DANIEL K. RESNICK, MD, MS
Professor and Vice Chairman, Program
Director, Department of Neurosurgery,
University of Wisconsin-Madison School of
Medicine and Public Health, Madison,
Wisconsin, USA

EDITORS

NATHANIEL P. BROOKS, MD, FAANS
Associate Professor, Department of
Neurological Surgery, University of Wisconsin,
Madison, Wisconsin, USA

MICHAEL Y. WANG, MD
Professor, Department of Neurological
Surgery, University of Miami Miller School of
Medicine, Miami, Florida, USA

AUTHORS

SANJAY BHATIA, MBBS, MCh, FAANS
Associate Professor, Department of
Neurosurgery, West Virginia University,
Morgantown, West Virginia, USA

NATHANIEL P. BROOKS, MD, FAANS
Associate Professor, Department of
Neurological Surgery, University of Wisconsin,
Madison, Wisconsin, USA

G. DAMIAN BRUSKO, BS
Department of Neurological Surgery, University
of Miami Miller School of Medicine, Lois Pope
Life Center, Miami, Florida, USA

MOHAMAD BYDON, MD
Mayo Clinic Neuro-Informatics Laboratory,
Department of Neurologic Surgery, Mayo
Clinic, Rochester, Minnesota, USA

VIKRAM CHAKRAVARTHY, MD
Chief Resident, Department of Neurosurgery,
Cleveland Clinic Lerner College of Medicine of
Case Western Reserve University, Cleveland
Clinic, Cleveland, Ohio, USA

DANIEL COUGHLIN, MD
Spine Fellow, Center for Spine Health,
Cleveland Clinic, Cleveland, Ohio, USA

CLAY M. ELSWICK, MD
Fellow, Department of Neurosurgery,
University of Michigan, Ann Arbor, Michigan,
USA

JACOB J. ENDERS, BS
Medical Student, Cleveland Clinic Lerner
College of Medicine, Cleveland Clinic,
Cleveland, Ohio, USA

ALEXANDRA M. GIANTINI-LARSEN, MD
Department of Neurological Surgery,
NewYork-Presbyterian Hospital/Weill Cornell
Medical Center, New York, New York, USA

ANSHIT GOYAL, MBBS
Mayo Clinic Neuro-Informatics Laboratory,
Department of Neurologic Surgery, Mayo
Clinic, Rochester, Minnesota, USA

MUHAMED HADZIPASIC, MD, PhD
Department of Neurosurgery, Massachusetts
General Hospital, Harvard Medical School,
Boston, Massachusetts, USA

SAQIB HASAN, MD
Attending Surgeon, Webster Orthopedics
Spine Institute, Oakland, California, USA

CHRISTOPH HOFSTETTER, MD, PhD
Associate Professor, Department of Neurological Surgery, University of Washington, Seattle, Washington, USA

WELLINGTON K. HSU, MD
Professor and Director of Research, Northwestern Department of Orthopedic Surgery, Chicago, Illinois, USA

JACOB R. JOSEPH, MD
Resident, Department of Neurosurgery, University of Michigan, Ann Arbor, Michigan, USA

MARTIN KOMP, MD
Center for Spine Surgery and Pain Therapy, Center for Orthopaedics and Traumatology of the St. Elisabeth Group–Catholic Hospitals Rhein-Ruhr, St. Anna Hospital Herne/Marien Hospital Herne University Hospital/Marien Hospital Witten, Herne, Germany

AJIT A. KRISHNANEY, MD, FAANS
Vice Chair, Department of Neurosurgery, Cleveland Clinic, Cleveland, Ohio, USA

MARIEL R. MANLAPAZ, MD
Director, Perioperative Medicine Fellowship, Department of General Anesthesia, Cleveland Clinic, Cleveland, Ohio, USA

DAVID J. MAZUR-HART, MD, MS
Resident, Department of Neurological Surgery, Oregon Health & Science University, Center for Health & Healing, Portland, Oregon, USA

ALI MOBASHERI, BSc, ARCS, MSc, DPhil (Oxon)
Department of Regenerative Medicine, State Research Institute Centre for Innovative Medicine, Vilnius, Lithuania; Research Unit of Medical Imaging, Physics and Technology, Faculty of Medicine, University of Oulu, Oulu, Finland; Sheik Salem Bin Mahfouz Scientific Chair, Centre for Sport, Exercise and Osteoarthritis Research Versus Arthritis, Queen's Medical Centre, Nottingham, United Kingdom; Treatment of Osteoarthritis with Stem Cells, King Abdulaziz University, Jeddah, Kingdom of Saudi Arabia

THOMAS E. MROZ, MD
Director, Center for Spine Health, Cleveland Clinic, Cleveland, Ohio, USA

MARK OPPENLANDER, MD
Assistant Professor, Department of Neurosurgery, University of Michigan, Ann Arbor, Michigan, USA

DANIEL E. OYON, MD
Department of Neurosurgery, Northwestern University Feinberg School of Medicine, Chicago, Illinois, USA

PAUL PARK, MD
Professor, Neurological Surgery, Department of Neurosurgery, University of Michigan, Ann Arbor, Michigan, USA

SHEERAZ QURESHI, MD, MBA
Associate Professor, Orthopaedic Surgery, Minimally Invasive Spinal Surgery, Hospital for Special Surgery, Weill Cornell Medical College, New York, New York, USA

STEPHEN M. RICHARDSON, BSc, PhD
Division of Cell Matrix Biology and Regenerative Medicine, School of Biological Sciences, Faculty of Biology, Medicine and Health, University of Manchester, Manchester Academic Health Sciences Centre, Manchester, United Kingdom

SEBASTIAN RUETTEN, MD
Center for Spine Surgery and Pain Therapy, Center for Orthopaedics and Traumatology of the St. Elisabeth Group–Catholic Hospitals Rhein-Ruhr, St. Anna Hospital Herne/Marien Hospital Herne University Hospital/Marien Hospital Witten, Herne, Germany

YAMAAN SAADEH, MD
Department of Neurosurgery, University of Michigan, Ann Arbor, Michigan, USA

ERIC SCHMIDT, MD
Department of Neurosurgery, Cleveland Clinic Lerner College of Medicine of Case Western Reserve University, Cleveland, Ohio, USA

VIVEK P. SHAH, BS
Research Assistant, Department of Orthopedic Surgery – Hsu Lab, Northwestern University, Chicago, Illinois, USA

SHEHRYAR SHEIKH, BA
Department of Neurosurgery, Cleveland Clinic
Lerner College of Medicine of Case Western
Reserve University, Cleveland, Ohio, USA

JOHN H. SHIN, MD
Department of Neurosurgery, Massachusetts
General Hospital, Harvard Medical School,
Boston, Massachusetts, USA

SANANTHAN SIVAKANTHAN, MD
Resident, Department of Neurological Surgery,
University of Washington, Seattle, Washington,
USA

JEREMY STEINBERGER, MD
Clinical Fellow, Hospital for Special Surgery,
New York, New York, USA

MICHAEL STEINMETZ, MD
Department of Neurosurgery, Cleveland
Clinic Lerner College of Medicine of Case
Western Reserve University, Cleveland,
Ohio, USA

MICHAEL J. STRONG, MD, PhD, MPH
Resident, Department of Neurosurgery,
University of Michigan, Ann Arbor, Michigan,
USA

HOUTAN A. TABA, MD
Spine Surgery Fellow, Department of
Orthopedics and Rehabilitation, University
of Wisconsin-Madison, Madison, Wisconsin,
USA

CLAUDIO E. TATSUI, MD
Department of Neurosurgery, Division of
Surgery, The University of Texas MD Anderson
Cancer Center, Houston, Texas, USA

KHOI D. THAN, MD
Assistant Professor, Department
of Neurological Surgery, Oregon
Health & Science University, Center for
Health & Healing, Portland, Oregon, USA

S. JOY TRYBULA, PharmD, MD
Department of Neurosurgery, Northwestern
University Feinberg School of Medicine,
Chicago, Illinois, USA

JUAN S. URIBE, MD, FAANS
Chief, Division of Spinal Disorders, Professor
and Vice Chair, Department of Neurosurgery,
Barrow Neurological Institute, St. Joseph's
Hospital and Medical Center, Phoenix, Arizona,
USA

SHALEEN VIRA, MD
Spine Fellow, Center for Spine Health,
Cleveland Clinic, Cleveland, Ohio, USA

MICHAEL Y. WANG, MD
Professor, Department of Neurological
Surgery, University of Miami Miller School of
Medicine, Miami, Florida, USA

JOSHUA T. WEWEL, MD
Department of Neurosurgery, Barrow
Neurological Institute, St. Joseph's Hospital
and Medical Center, Phoenix, Arizona, USA

SETH K. WILLIAMS, MD
Associate Professor, Vice Chair of Clinical
Operations, Department of Orthopedics and
Rehabilitation, University of Wisconsin-
Madison, Madison, Wisconsin, USA

JEAN-PAUL WOLINSKY, MD
Professor of Neurosurgery and Orthopaedic
Surgery, Vice Chairman of Neurosurgery -
Strategic Planning and Finance, Director of
Spinal Oncology, Department of Neurosurgery,
Northwestern University Feinberg School of
Medicine, Chicago, Illinois, USA

HANA YOKOI, BS
Case Western Reserve University School of
Medicine, Cleveland, Ohio, USA

YAGIZ U. YOLCU, MD
Mayo Clinic Neuro-Informatics Laboratory,
Department of Neurologic Surgery, Mayo
Clinic, Rochester, Minnesota, USA

SHEHRYAR BHESGI, DA.
Department of Neurosurgery, Cleveland Clinic Lerner College of Medicine of Case Western Reserve University, Cleveland, Ohio, USA

JOHN H. SHIM, MD
Department of Neurosurgery, ...

JEREMY STEINBERGER, MD
Clinical Fellow, Hospital for Special Surgery, New York, New York, USA

MICHAEL STEINMETZ, MD
Department of Neurosurgery, Cleveland Clinic Lerner College of Medicine of Case Western Reserve University, Cleveland, Ohio, USA

MICHAEL J. STRONG, MD, PhD, MPH
Resident, Department of Neurosurgery, University of Michigan, Ann Arbor, Michigan, USA

HOUMAN A. TABA, MD
Spine Surgery Fellow, Department of Orthopaedics and Rehabilitation, University of Wisconsin-Madison, Madison, Wisconsin, USA

CLAUDIO E. TATSUI, MD
Department of Neurosurgery, Division of Surgery, The University of Texas MD Anderson Cancer Center, Houston, Texas, USA

KHOI D. THAN, MD
Assistant Professor, Department of Neurological Surgery, Oregon Health & Science University, Center for ..., Portland, Oregon, USA

S. JOY TRYBULA, MD
Department of Neurosurgery, Northwestern University Feinberg School of Medicine, Chicago, Illinois, USA

JUAN S. URIBE, MD, FAANS
Chief, Division of Spinal Disorders, Professor ...

... VIRK, MD
...Spine Center for Spine Health, Cleveland Clinic, Cleveland, Ohio, USA

MICHAEL Y. WANG, MD
Professor, Department of Neurological Surgery, University of Miami Miller School of Medicine, Miami, Florida, USA

JOSHUA T. WEWEL, MD
Department of Neurosurgery, Barrow Neurological Institute, St. Joseph's Hospital and Medical Center, Phoenix, Arizona, USA

SETH K. WILLIAMS, MD
Associate Professor, Vice Chair of Clinical Operations, Department of Orthopaedics and Rehabilitation, University of Wisconsin, Madison, Wisconsin, USA

JEAN-PAUL WOLINSKY, MD
Professor of Neurosurgery and Orthopaedic Surgery, Vice Chairman of Neurosurgery, Strategic Planning and Finance, Director of Spinal Oncology, Department of Neurosurgery, Northwestern University Feinberg School of Medicine, Chicago, Illinois, USA

HANA YOKOL, BS
Case Western Reserve University School of Medicine, Cleveland, Ohio, USA

YAGIZ U. YOLCU, MD
Mayo Clinic Neuro-Informatics Laboratory, Department of Neurologic Surgery, Mayo Clinic, Rochester, Minnesota, USA

Contents

> Full-endoscopic spine surgery has been developed to decrease approach-related morbidity and provide superior visualization. Using a working channel endoscope, lumbar disc herniations can be approached via two complementary corridors: the transforaminal approach and the interlaminar approach. Indications, contraindications, surgical technique, complications, and outcomes are discussed in this article. Multiple published studies have demonstrated the feasibility, safety, and efficacy of full-endoscopic lumbar discectomies. Emerging evidence suggests that full-endoscopic discectomies result in similar functional outcomes compared with microsurgical technique and are associated with shorter hospital stays, less opioid consumption, and fewer perioperative complications.

 Video content accompanies this article at http://www.neurosurgery.theclinics.com.

> Unilateral cervical nerve root compression causing radiculopathy, which does not improve with conservative measures, is safely and effectively treated with surgery. Both anterior and posterior approaches have been described. Overall results from either of these broad categories of approaches are equivalent. Posterior approaches target the cervical root compression directly and allow decompression by widening the neural foramen and/or removing a lateral disc fragment. Following success of the open technique, variations of this technique were introduced to minimize approach-related complications.

> Spine surgeons have recently developed more advanced and less invasive techniques. One significant example of recent surgical innovation is the advent of endoscopic-assisted spine surgery. Endoscopic lumbar interbody fusions are increasingly used to treat lumbar degenerative disease in a minimally invasive approach that minimizes pain and maximizes outcomes. Numerous technical refinements to ultraminimally invasive approaches have occurred since their initial use, which has resulted in substantial clinical benefit for patients that remains stable over time. Serious complications can occur and thus, the spine surgeon adopting endoscopic techniques must be aware of the early learning curve.

The most common causes of degenerative narrowing of the spinal canal are disc herniations and spinal canal stenosis. The standard surgical procedure for lumbar spinal canal stenosis today is microsurgical, microscope-assisted decompression. Full-endoscopic decompression is now also technically feasible and more widespread because of the development of surgical access techniques and instruments. The use of the different access technique depends on the anatomic and pathologic inclusion and exclusion criteria. Sufficient decompression can now be achieved using full-endoscopic techniques in a standardized minimally invasive procedure. This article describes the technique for the full-endoscopic decompression of the lumbar spine.

Lateral lumbar interbody fusion (LLIF) is a minimally invasive technique that allows access to the lumbar spine from L1/2 to L4/5 for placement of wide interbody devices. This technique is used in the treatment of degenerative conditions, deformity, and infectious, neoplastic, and traumatic thoracolumbar pathology. LLIF allows placement of interbody devices across the apophysis, which leads to powerful coronal deformity correction and indirect decompression from restoration of disk height. Literature shows equivalent to superior outcomes of the LLIF technique to anterior or posterior techniques in the treatment of degenerative conditions while avoiding the complications associated with larger procedures.

The lateral retropleural thoracic approach offers minimally invasive access for the treatment of thoracic spine pathology, specifically thoracic herniated discs. Alternatives to the retropleural approach traditionally included posterolateral or anterior approaches, which carry increased morbidity. The retropleural approach affords lateral access to the thoracic spine that allows for addressing pathology such as herniated discs, corpectomy, tumor, or trauma. This article outlines preoperative workup and planning, intraoperative steps, tips, and postoperative care.

Surgical procedures, such as spinal fusion and disk replacement, are commonly used for treatment following failure of conservative treatment in degenerative spine disease. However, there is growing consensus that currently available surgical technologies may have long-term inefficacy for successful management. Intervertebral disk degeneration is the most common manifestation of degenerative spine disease, hence, replacement/repair of this tissue is an important component of surgical treatment. Restoration of spinal alignment and preservation of natural kinematics is also essential to a good outcome. This article reviews novel intervertebral implant technologies that have the potential to significantly impact elective spine surgery for degenerative spine disease.

Patients with symptomatic instability of the spine may be treated surgically with interbody fusion. Cost and complexity in this procedure arises owing to the implanted materials involved with facilitating fusion such as titanium or polyetheretherketone. Surface modifications have been developed to augment these base materials such as plasma-spraying polyetheretherketone with titanium or coating implants with hydroxyapatite. Although some evidence has been gathered on these novel materials, additional study is needed to establish the true efficacy of surface modifications for interbody fusion devices in improving long-term patient outcomes.

There are a number of bone regeneration therapeutics available to aid spinal fusion; however, many are associated with pseudarthrosis, inflammation, and other complications. Mesenchymal stem cells for fusion has been promoted to mitigate these risks and achieve successful bony fusion. This article reviews the clinical studies available with use in spinal fusion. Preliminary results demonstrate that stem cells can provide high rates of fusion, comparable to autograft, without associated morbidity. Autologous and allogeneic stem cell sources showed similar rates of fusion in this review. Further research is required to evaluate which clinical situations are the optimum for stem cell use.

Anterior cervical disc replacement (arthroplasty) has gained momentum over the past 2 decades. The ball-and-socket prosthesis design of arthroplasty has been shown to simulate normal motion in all 3 rotation planes at the level of surgery and replicates physiologic motion. Anterior cervical discectomy and fusion has been shown to be a safe and effective surgery over decades; cervical disc replacement counters some secondary effects owing to its preservation of segmental mobility, the potential to reduce adjacent segment degeneration, and the lack of plating or harvesting bone graft. The literature is growing in support of the success and longevity of arthroplasty.

Enhanced recovery after surgery is an interdisciplinary, multimodal approach to improve postoperative outcomes by applying multiple evidenced-based interventions. It has been adapted at multiple institutions for patients undergoing spine surgery to combat the rising rate of opioid consumption. Various preoperative, intraoperative, and postoperative pharmacologic and nonpharmacologic interventions have been introduced to augment patient care with the goal to decrease hospital length of stay and improve postoperative outcomes. Future studies will focus on health care-related quality of life outcomes to evaluate the effectiveness of enhanced recovery after surgery across various benchmarks.

NEUROSURGERY CLINICS OF NORTH AMERICA

SERIES OF RELATED INTEREST

Neurologic Clinics
http://www.neurologicclinics.com
Neuroimaging Clinics
http://www.neuroimaging.theclinics.com/

THE CLINICS ARE AVAILABLE ONLINE!
Access your subscription at:
www.theclinics.com

Preface
New Technologies in Spine Surgery

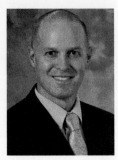
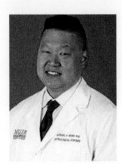

Nathaniel P. Brooks, MD   Michael Y. Wang, MD

Editors

The techniques and technologies employed in spine surgery are in a continuous state of evolution because surgeons, scientists, and patients are in a constant quest for technologies that will allow easier, less painful surgery with faster recoveries. The ideal technologies would allow painless procedures, requiring no recovery and reversing the effects of disease. Have we achieved these goals? No. Are we closer to these goals than we were 20 years ago? 50 years? Yes and yes. This issue of *Neurosurgery Clinics of North America* includes a collection of articles from world-renowned experts describing the newest technologies and techniques to help patients achieve these goals. The articles span the continuum from surface technologies to endoscopic surgical approaches to robotics. Please read on to learn how these technologies can benefit your patients.

Nathaniel P. Brooks, MD
Department of Neurological Surgery
University of Wisconsin–Madison
600 Highland Avenue, CSC K4/860
Madison, WI 53792, USA

Michael Y. Wang, MD
Department of Neurological Surgery
University of Miami
Miller School of Medicine
1095 NW 14th Terrace
Miami, FL 33136, USA

E-mail addresses:
brooks@neurosurgery.wisc.edu (N.P. Brooks)
mwang2@med.miami.edu (M.Y. Wang)

Full-Endoscopic Lumbar Discectomy

Sananthan Sivakanthan, MD[a], Saqib Hasan, MD[b], Christoph Hofstetter, MD, PhD[a],*

KEYWORDS

- Full-endoscopic spine surgery • Lumbar discectomy
- Interlaminar endoscopic lumbar discectomy (IELD)
- Transforaminal endoscopic lumbar discectomy (TELD)

KEY POINTS

- Full-endoscopic spine surgery allows treatment of the vast majority of lumbar disc herniations.
- Lumbar disc herniations may be approached via a transforaminal or interlaminar corridor.
- Full-endoscopic discectomies lead to functional outcomes similar to microdiscectomies
- Full-endoscopic discectomies are associated with fewer perioperative complications compared to microdiscectomies

INTRODUCTION

Lumbar disc herniation is a posterior displacement of either the nucleus pulposus or the annulus fibrosis (or both) beyond the intervertebral space. Disc herniations may compress spinal nerve roots which can lead to symptomatic lumbar radiculopathy, a major cause of morbidity and cost. The prevalence of symptomatic lumbar disc disease is estimated to range from 1% to 2% in the United States.[1] Spontaneous regression of lumbar disc herniations occurs in most patients. Accordingly, 60% to 90% of patients are treated successfully with conservative treatment strategies.[2] Non-operative therapy typically constitutes the first-line treatment and consists of physical therapy, non-steroidal medications, and epidural steroid injections. Only if patients do not improve after a 4- to 8-week trial of non-operative therapy, is surgery recommended. Exceptions, of course, are made for patients with progressive neurologic deficits or cauda equina syndrome. Surgical treatment of lumbar disc herniations results in better pain relief, less back pain-related disability, and better return of function compared with conservative therapy.[3]

The first operation for a ruptured intervertebral disc was carried out by Mixter and Barr in 1932.[4] A complete laminectomy was performed and a large disc fragment was resected transdurally. Later, a more minimal bone removal and extradural discectomy was proposed by Love and Walsh.[5] Surgical technique was further refined by the introduction of the operative microscope by Yasargil and colleagues.[6] Tubular retractors splitting the paraspinal muscle instead of cutting them were introduced to minimize retractor-related soft tissue trauma.[7] Tubular retractors were equipped with integrated endoscopes to facilitate visualization of the pathology.[8,9] A full-endoscopic interlaminar technique was made possible with the development of efficient working channel endoscopes, efficient burrs, and rongeurs.[10,11]

Transforaminal access was developed based on previous non-visualized percutaneous indirect spinal canal decompression via the medial aspect of the foraminal annular window (Kambin's triangle).[12,13] The first endoscopic visualization of the herniated nucleus pulposus was published by Kambin and colleagues[14] in 1988. The development of the YESS working channel endoscope

[a] Department of Neurological Surgery, University of Washington, Seattle, WA, USA; [b] Webster Orthopedics Spine Institute, Oakland, CA, USA
* Corresponding author. Campus Box 356470, Room RR734, 1959 Northeast Pacific Street, Seattle, WA 98195-6470.
E-mail address: chh9045@uw.edu

Neurosurg Clin N Am 31 (2020) 1–7
https://doi.org/10.1016/j.nec.2019.08.016
1042-3680/20/© 2019 Elsevier Inc. All rights reserved.

allowed for the first endoscopically visualized discectomies via the transforaminal route.[15] Widening of the foraminal window by removing the ventral portion of the superior articular process with bone reamers enabled safe transforaminal access in almost all instances.[16]

TRANSFORAMINAL ENDOSCOPIC LUMBAR DISCECTOMY
Indications/Contraindications

The endoscopic transforaminal approach allows for resection of disc herniations located in the foramen or in the lateral recess *ventral to the traversing nerve root*. This approach is most applicable to spinal segments cephalad to L5/S1. It also allows access to central disc herniations. Relative contraindications to transforaminal endoscopic lumbar discectomy (TELD) include severe foraminal stenosis, facet hypertrophy, and location of the exiting nerve root within the inferior portion of the foramen. In these cases, a trans-superior articular process approach is recommended. Extensive migration of the disc sequester also constitutes a relative contraindication because it requires modification of the transforaminal approach. Spinal instability or severe scoliosis (>40°) are absolute contraindications.

Surgical Technique

1. Sedation
   - Either general endotracheal anesthesia or conscious sedation.
2. Patient positioning
   - Either prone on a Jackson table with a Wilson frame or in lateral decubitus position with the symptomatic side up.
3. Plan approach trajectory and incision
   - Estimate the necessary distance of the skin incision from the midline on pre-operative axial T2-weighted MRI studies. As a general guideline, the distance is approximately:
     o 8 cm at L3/4.
     o 10 cm at L4/5
     o 12 cm at L5/S1 (**Fig. 1**A)
   - Adjust the distance to the midline by referencing to the lateral projection of the spinous process on a lateral radiograph. For a typical transforaminal approach, the skin incision is in the vicinity of the tip of the spinous process (**Fig. 1**B).
   - Determine the rostrocaudal inclination to allow for a trans-isthmic approach to the lesion to be treated. Typically, the inclination is 20° to 30° (**Fig. 1**C, d).
4. Imaging-palpation-visualization of target area

- An 18G needle is advanced toward the medial aspect of the foraminal annular window (Kambin's triangle, *target area*). Typically, the lateral aspect of the facet joint is palpated first and the needle is then "walked" ventrally along the lateral aspect of the superior articular process toward Kambin's triangle. Appropriate position of the needle tip is confirmed on anteroposterior (AP) and lateral radiographs (**Fig. 2**).
- The endoscope is brought in and the content of Kambin's triangle is visualized.
5. Perform foraminoplasty using a burr
   - The ventral aspect of the superior articular process can be resected, if necessary, to gain access to the lesion.
6. Direct visualization of the principal anatomic landmark
   - The caudal index level pedicle serves as the *principal anatomic landmark* and is directly visualized and confirmed on an AP radiograph (**Fig. 3**).
7. Identify the traversing nerve root
   - Rostral and medial to the caudal pedicle the traversing nerve root is identified.
8. Resection of disc sequester
   - The disc sequester is visualized, mobilized with the radiofrequency probe and resected using grasping forceps (**Fig. 4**A, B).
9. Visually confirm decompression of neural elements (**Fig. 4**C)

Complications and Management

- Intraoperative dural tears can occur, particularly in upper lumbar segments, and may be caused by bone reamers. To avoid postoperative radiculopathies, dural lacerations should be treated with DuraGen inlay grafts and sealed with Tisseel.
- Retained disc fragments—this is commonly due to inadequate foraminoplasty not allowing visualization of the principal anatomic landmark and neural elements.
- Postoperative paresthesias occur from intraoperative irritation of the exiting nerve root and occur on postoperative day 3. They typically respond to nonsteroidal anti-inflammatory drugs and gabapentin. Severe cases may be treated with a transforaminal steroid injection.

INTERLAMINAR ENDOSCOPIC LUMBAR DISCECTOMY
Indications/Contraindications

The endoscopic interlaminar approach is well suited for resection of subarticular disc herniations, particularly in the lower lumbar segment

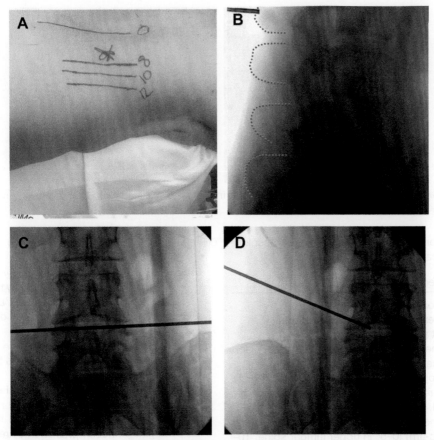

Fig. 1. For orientation, three vertical lines 8, 10, 12 cm off midline are marked on the patient before draping (*A*). The pre-determined distance from the midline is referenced to the lateral projection of the tip of the spinous processes (*blue dotted line*) (*B*). The AP projection of index disc space is marked on an AP endplate view (*C*). The rostrocaudal inclination of the approach trajectory is estimated by connecting the rostral aspect of the superior articular process and the medial aspect of the foraminal annular window (target area, *D*).

(L4/5 and L5/S1). This approach is particularly useful in cases of subarticular disc herniations and concomitant lateral recess stenosis. Relative contraindications for interlaminar endoscopic lumbar discectomy (IELD) include previous posterior surgery, location in the upper lumbar levels, or extensive facet overgrowth. In some of these cases TELD should be considered. Spinal

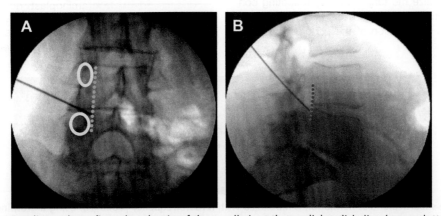

Fig. 2. An AP radiograph confirms that the tip of the needle is at the medial pedicle line (*green dotted line*, *A*). On lateral radiograph the tip of the needle remains behind the posterior vertebral line (*red dotted line*, *B*).

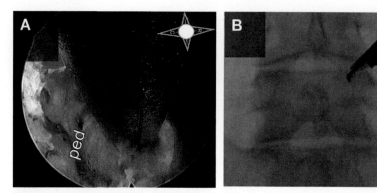

Fig. 3. Visualize the caudal index level pedicle (ped, principal anatomic landmark, *A*) and confirm on AP fluoroscopic image (*B*).

instability or severe scoliosis (>40°) are absolute contraindications.

Surgical Technique

1. Sedation
   - General endotracheal anesthesia.
2. Patient positioning
   - Prone on a Jackson table with a Wilson frame.
3. Plan approach trajectory
   - Obtain AP endplate view of the caudal index level.
   - For non-migrated disc herniations caudal tilt the c-arm (0–5° in upper lumbar spine, 10–15° in lower lumbar spine) to center the gap between the spinous process on the disc space (**Fig. 5**)
   - Adjust trajectory as needed for migrated disc sequesters
4. Imaging-palpation-visualization of the target area
   - Identify the *target area* (inferomedial edge of the lamina) on fluoroscopic imaging (**Fig. 6**A).
   - Palpate the target area with a trocar (**Fig. 6**B).
   - Visualize the target area by resecting connecting tissue (**Fig. 6**C).
5. Direct visualization of the principal anatomic landmark

   - Visualize the yellow ligament (*principal anatomic landmark*).
6. Medial facetectomy
   - A medial facetectomy is typically necessary at spinal segments cephalad to L5/S1 and carried out with a high-speed drill and a Kerrison rongeur.
7. Enter the epidural space
   - Use a micro punch to transgress the yellow ligament (**Fig. 7**)
8. Identify the lateral margin of neural elements
9. Resection of disc sequester
   - Disc sequesters visible beyond the lateral margins of the neural elements are retrieved (**Fig. 8**A).
10. Retraction of neural elements
    - Medialize the neural elements with a blunt dissector.
    - Advance the working cannula into the spinal canal (bevel facing medially).
    - Rotate the working cannula 180°.
11. Resect residual/contained disc fragments and explore the annular defect (**Fig. 8**B)

Complications and Management

- Intraoperative dural tears can occur, particularly in revision cases. To avoid postoperative radiculopathies they should be treated with

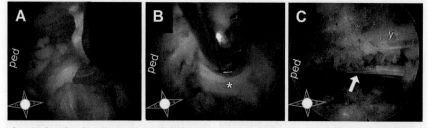

Fig. 4. The subarticular disc herniation is mobilized with a radiofrequency probe (*A*). Using a grasping forceps, the fragment is retrieved (*B*). Following the discectomy complete decompression of the traversing nerve root (*arrow*) is visualized (*C*).

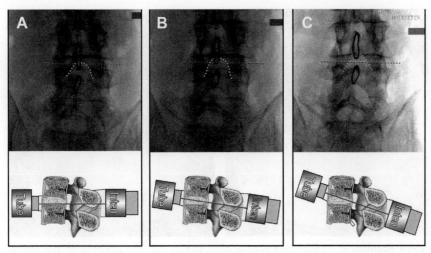

Fig. 5. Adjustment of the c-arm for the interlaminar approach. First an AP endplate view of the superior endplate of the caudal index level is obtained (L3/4, *green arrowheads, A*). The addition of distal tilt to the rostrocaudal X-ray beam angle moves the projection of the superior spinous process space rostrally (*arrowhead, B*). Once the gap between spinous processes is centered over the projection of the disc space an ideal rostrocaudal trajectory has been determined (*arrowhead, C*). Note the inferior edge of the rostral index lamina (*red dotted line*), which serves as a docking point for the trocar during the approach.

DuraGen inlay grafts and sealed with Tisseel. In cases of dural defects too large for inlay grafts conversion to open surgery for primary repair should be considered.
- Intraoperative bleeding:
  - Meticulous surgical technique and use of a radiofrequency probe
  - Increase the continuous irrigation pressure (however, irrigation pressure is recommended to be maintained below the systemic diastolic blood pressure)
  - Supplement irrigation fluid with 1 mg of epinephrine/3 L bag
- Postoperative hematomas with neurologic deficits
  - The decision to return to the operating room is a clinical decision because immediate postoperative MRIs are typically not useful to determine the degree of compression. A

stat MRI is then obtained to determine the location and possible expansion of the hematoma, which informs the decision on what technique to use. A small localized hematoma in the resection cavity can be washed out with full-endoscopic technique. A hematoma which has expanded epidurally will require a more traditional surgical approach.
- Recurrent disc herniation after IELD.
  - A transforaminal approach should be considered because it avoids postoperative scar tissue.

POSTOPERATIVE CARE FOR INTERLAMINAR AND TRANSFORAMINAL ENDOSCOPIC LUMBAR DISCECTOMY

Patients are typically discharged on the same day of the procedure. Routine follow-up is needed to

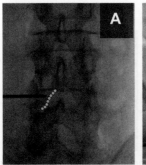
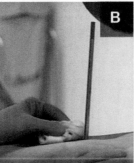
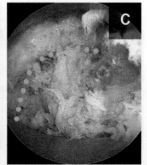

Fig. 6. Identify the target area (inferomedial edge of the lamina, *green dotted line*) on fluoroscopic imaging (*A*). Palpate target area with trocar (*B*). Visualize the target area (*green dotted line*) by resecting attached soft tissue (*C*).

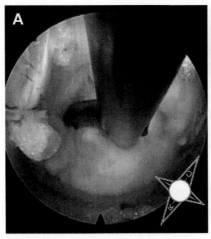
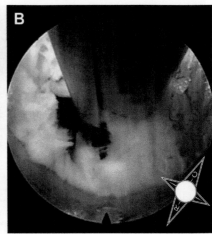

Fig. 7. The yellow ligament is transgressed with a micro-punch (*A*). The opening of the yellow ligament is enlarged using a Kerrison rongeur (*B*).

assess for improvement in symptomatology. Lack of improvement is typically seen if the surgery was based on an incorrect pre-operative diagnosis. Recurrence of pain may suggest a re-herniation and should prompt re-imaging, particularly if it is associated with recurrent or new neurologic deficits.

OUTCOMES FOR INTERLAMINAR AND TRANSFORAMINAL ENDOSCOPIC LUMBAR DISCECTOMY

There is an abundance of literature supporting the use of full-endoscopic spine surgery for performing lumbar discectomies. Several randomized controlled and prospective studies have investigated clinical outcomes following full endoscopic microdiscectomy.[17–19] Ruetten at al.[17] conducted a prospective controlled study of 200 patients who were randomized to either full-endoscopic discectomy (transforaminal or interlaminar) or open microsurgical discectomy with 2-year follow-up. Both groups experienced similar improvements in pain and function; however, a statistically significant number of patients in the microsurgical group experienced greater back pain postoperatively. There were no significant differences in re-operation rates between the two groups; however, the endoscopic cohort was found to have statistically significant fewer complications, less postoperative pain medication requirements, and less postoperative work disability. Similarly, Gibson and colleagues[18] conducted a prospective randomized controlled study of 140 patients who underwent endoscopic transforaminal discectomies or open microsurgical discectomy with 2-year follow-up available on 123 patients. Although both cohorts noted significant improvement from baseline, VAS leg pain scores at 2 years were significantly less following endoscopic discectomy (1.9 ± 2.6) when compared with microsurgical discectomy (3.5 ± 3.1, $P = .002$). There was no significant difference in reoperation and complication rates between the cohorts; however, the endoscopic group was found to have a significantly shorter length of hospital stay. Lastly, Chen and colleagues[19] conducted a prospective randomized study including 80 TELD versus 73

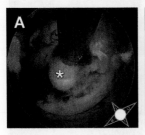
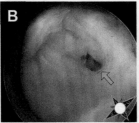
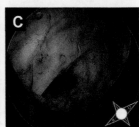

Fig. 8. Disc sequesters (*asterisk*) are retrieved using grasping forceps using an alligator movement which allows to monitor the dura (*A*). On retraction of the neural elements, the annular defect (*green arrow*) is explored and loose disc fragments are retrieved (*B*). The traversing nerve root is inspected following decompression (*C*).

microsurgical discectomies. In this study, 1-year follow-up data were available in 137 patients. The study found that improvement of leg pain and back disability was similar following TELD and microsurgical discectomy at 1-year follow-up. There was a tendency toward a lower rate of complications in TELD (13.8%) compared with microsurgical discectomies (16.4%); however, this did not reach statistical significance. In conclusion, full-endoscopic surgery achieves similar functional outcomes compared with microsurgical discectomies with a reduction of perioperative complications.

SUMMARY

Full-endoscopic lumbar discectomy is an innovative, minimally invasive alternative to microdiscectomy for patients with symptomatic lumbar disc herniations. IELD and TELD offer two complementary surgical corridors to spinal pathology and allow for treatment of the vast majority of lumbar disc herniations. There is level one evidence suggesting that full-endoscopic spine surgery results in similar functional outcomes compared with microsurgical technique, and has a favorable rate of perioperative complications.

ACKNOWLEDGMENTS

This work was generously supported by the Raisbeck family foundation.

REFERENCES

1. Deyo RA, Tsui-Wu YJ. Descriptive epidemiology of low-back pain and its related medical care in the United States. Spine (Phila Pa 1976) 1987;12(3): 264–8.
2. Chiu CC, Chuang TY, Chang KH, et al. The probability of spontaneous regression of lumbar herniated disc: a systematic review. Clin Rehabil 2015;29(2): 184–95.
3. Chen BL, Guo JB, Zhang HW, et al. Surgical versus non-operative treatment for lumbar disc herniation: a systematic review and meta-analysis. Clin Rehabil 2018;32(2):146–60.
4. Mixter W, Barr J. Rupture of the intervertebral disc with involvement of the spinal canal. N Engl J Med 1932;211:210–5.
5. Love J, Walsh M. Protruded intervertebral disks. Report of one hundred cases in which operation was performed. JAMA 1938;111:396–400.
6. Yasargil MG, Vise WM, Bader DC. Technical adjuncts in neurosurgery. Surg Neurol 1977;8(5): 331–6.
7. Foley KT. Microendoscopic discectomy. Tech Neurosurg 1997;3:301–7.
8. Perez-Cruet MJ, Foley KT, Isaacs RE, et al. Microendoscopic lumbar discectomy: technical note. Neurosurgery 2002;51(5 Suppl):S129–36.
9. Nakagawa H, Kamimura M, Uchiyama S, et al. Microendoscopic discectomy (MED) for lumbar disc prolapse. J Clin Neurosci 2003;10(2):231–5.
10. Choi G, Lee SH, Raiturker PP, et al. Percutaneous endoscopic interlaminar discectomy for intracanalicular disc herniations at L5-S1 using a rigid working channel endoscope. Neurosurgery 2006;58(1 Suppl):ONS59–68 [discussion: ONS59–68].
11. Ruetten S, Komp M, Merk H, et al. Use of newly developed instruments and endoscopes: full-endoscopic resection of lumbar disc herniations via the interlaminar and lateral transforaminal approach. J Neurosurg Spine 2007;6(6):521–30.
12. Kambin P. Arthroscopic microdiscectomy: minimal intervention spinal surgery. Baltimore (MD): Urban & Schwarzenberg; 1990.
13. Hijikata S, Yamagishi M, Nakayma T. Percutaneous discectomy: a new treatment method for lumbar disc herniation. J Toden Hosp 1975;5:5–13.
14. Kambin P, Nixon JE, Chait A, et al. Annular protrusion: pathophysiology and roentgenographic appearance. Spine (Phila Pa 1976) 1988;13(6): 671–5.
15. Yeung AT. The evolution and advancement of endoscopic foraminal surgery: one surgeon's experience incorporating adjunctive techologies. SAS J 2007; 1(3):108–17.
16. Schubert M, Hoogland T. Endoscopic transforaminal nucleotomy with foraminoplasty for lumbar disk herniation. Oper Orthop Traumatol 2005;17(6):641–61.
17. Ruetten S, Komp M, Merk H, et al. Full-endoscopic interlaminar and transforaminal lumbar discectomy versus conventional microsurgical technique: a prospective, randomized, controlled study. Spine (Phila Pa 1976) 2008;33(9):931–9.
18. Gibson JNA, Subramanian AS, Scott CEH. A randomised controlled trial of transforaminal endoscopic discectomy vs microdiscectomy. Eur Spine J 2017;26(3):847–56.
19. Chen Z, Zhang L, Dong J, et al. Percutaneous transforaminal endoscopic discectomy compared with microendoscopic discectomy for lumbar disc herniation: 1-year results of an ongoing randomized controlled trial. J Neurosurg Spine 2018;28(3): 300–10.

Posterior Endoscopic Cervical Foraminotomy

Sanjay Bhatia, MBBS, MCh[a], Nathaniel P. Brooks, MD[b],*

KEYWORDS

- Cervical radiculopathy • Cervical foraminal stenosis • Posterior cervical foraminotomy
- Minimally invasive surgery • Endoscopic foraminotomy • Fully endoscopic technique

KEY POINTS

- The posterior cervical endoscopic technique allows cervical foraminal decompression, which is clinically and radiologically similar to open techniques.
- Access-related complications are minimized and outcomes are comparable, to both anterior and other posterior techniques.
- The fully endoscopic technique has a learning curve. Visual cues and anatomic expectations cannot be easily translated over from open techniques.

 Video content accompanies this article at http://www.neurosurgery.theclinics.com.

INTRODUCTION

Cervical radicular pain is a common condition that arises from lateral disc herniations or degenerative narrowing of the cervical foramina. Surgical decompression is often successful when conservative measures fail to relieve pain or if there is significant weakness in the muscles supplied by the affected root. Although anterior cervical discectomy and fusion (ACDF) continues to be a common treatment option, posterior approaches are becoming more commonly used, when the pathology being addressed is a lateral disc herniation or cervical foraminal stenosis, with equivalent results.[1–4] Cost-analysis studies favor posterior foraminotomy over ACDF.[5,6] Open foraminotomy,[1,7] minimally invasive foraminotomy (using a tube system with a microscope or endoscope),[8–11] as well as fully endoscopic techniques have been described.[12,13] No significant differences in clinical outcomes, complication rate, and reoperation rate have been demonstrated between posterior foraminotomies and ACDF for cervical radiculopathy.[14,15] One of the oft cited problems with posterior approaches has been axial neck pain that has been thought to result from injury to the paraspinal muscles.[16] Use of tubular retractors minimizes this damage and with the advent of newer endoscopic technology and equipment it has become possible to achieve the goals of posterior cervical foraminal discectomy/decompression, with minimal approach-related tissue damage. There is mixed data suggesting posterior approaches may contribute to the subsequent development of cervical kyphosis, especially for patients with preexisting loss of cervical lordosis (Cobb angle <10°).[17] Won and colleagues[16] evaluated this potential problem and found that posterior endoscopic foraminotomy was effective in reducing radicular symptoms and that preexisting loss of cervical lordosis (segmental Cobb angle <10°) did not lead to worse outcomes or increasing deformity.

This article describes the indications, equipment, technique, and complication avoidance of the fully endoscopic posterior cervical foraminotomy.

Disclosure Statement: The authors have nothing to disclose.

a Department of Neurosurgery, West Virginia University, One Medical Center Drive, Morgantown, WV 26506, USA; b Department of Neurological Surgery, University of Wisconsin, 600 Highland Avenue, K4/860, Madison, WI 53792, USA

* Corresponding author.

E-mail address: brooks@neurosurgery.wisc.edu

Neurosurg Clin N Am 31 (2020) 9–16
https://doi.org/10.1016/j.nec.2019.08.001
1042-3680/20/© 2019 Elsevier Inc. All rights reserved.

Clinical Indications

Posterior approaches are indicated for cervical radiculopathy, which has (1) failed conservative treatment and (2) is caused by either lateral disc herniation or foraminal stenosis from facet degeneration and osseoligamentous hypertrophy, as documented by imaging (computed tomographic myelogram, MRI). Selective nerve root blocks or electromyograms may be considered to assist in localization of the symptomatic level especially when the clinical level is equivocal and the imaging shows multilevel disease.

Anatomic Indications

The fully endoscopic approach is indicated for disc herniations that are mainly lateral to the edge of the thecal sac and do not extend significantly in a rostral or caudal direction. The disc herniation should not compress the spinal cord. The endoscopic posterior foraminotomy is not indicated in the following conditions: instability, significant deformity, presence of myelopathy, or cord compression and central canal stenosis, from central disc herniation or osteophytes.

Anatomy of the Cervical Foramina

The cervical foramina extend from the inferior aspect of the pedicle to the superior aspect of the pedicle of the inferior vertebrae. The anterior wall of the foramina is formed by the uncinate process, the posterolateral aspect of the intervertebral disc, and the adjoining vertebral body. The facet joint along with the superior articular process of the lower vertebra forms the posterior wall of the foramina. The nerve root enters the foramen medially at the medial border of the rostral and caudal pedicle and exits the foramen laterally as it passes the lateral margin of the rostral and caudal pedicles. In the sagittal oblique plane, the nerve roots are seen to lie below a line drawn from the tip of the uncinate process to the tip of the superior articular process.[18] In cadavers the nerve root is located more cranially in the foramen if the neck is fully extended.[19]

Endoscopic Equipment

The cervical endoscope system consists of a working sheath and an endoscope. The working sheath is a tubular retractor that is used to protect the intervening soft tissues and also can be used to dissect and retract. A variety of working sheaths with different length, diameters, and tip configuration are manufactured. The endoscope consists of a rod lens assembly, an irrigation channel; and a working channel through which instruments can be introduced and used. The optic view angle is typically 25 degrees. The outer diameter ranges from 5.9 × 5.0 mm to 6.9 × 5.6 mm. The working channel for the 5.9 mm scope is 3.1 mm and for the 6.9 mm scope it is 4.1 mm. The working channel is located eccentrically. The working length ranges from 124 to 205 mm. The endoscope is attached to a fiberoptic cable for light transmission, an irrigation system, and a camera. The images are visualized on a high-definition monitor. Various instruments are offered for use through the working channel. Forceps, rongeurs, dissectors, and bone punches of varying shapes and sizes are accessible. Flexible tip probes and radiofrequency bipolars are also available. Finally, a variety of powered drills and burrs are also available for use during the procedure. Accessories such as a fluid adapter may be used to increase the outflow resistance to the irrigation.

The endoscope provides illumination and magnification of the area of interest, the continuous irrigation keeps the surgical area clear for an unobstructed view, and the 25-degree angled field of view of the typical scope provides the ability to view a larger area along the margins of the working channel.

Posterior Endoscopic Cervical Foraminotomy Technique

Posterior endoscopic cervical foraminotomy (single or multilevel) is typically performed as an outpatient procedure (Video 1). The procedure is generally performed under general anesthesia, in the prone position. The senior author uses a 3-point bolster bed frame ("Jackson table"). The head is placed on a foam face support, with easily obtainable flexion, and taped down to maintain the position. The shoulders are also retracted caudally within physiologic limits with tape. Pins and rigid skull fixation may be used but are not generally required. The arms are positioned along the side of the body and all pressure points are padded. The head end of the table is elevated to reduce the pressure in epidural veins.

After preparation and draping of the field, fluoroscopy is performed to localize the level of interest and the laminar-facet junction (**Fig. 1**). A stab incision (~8–10 mm) is placed over the level of interest targeting the medial facet at the appropriate level. It is helpful to pierce the underlying fascia to allow the tissue dilator to pass more freely. A tissue dilator is then passed bluntly to the facet joint and lateral fluoroscopic images are obtained. The outer working sheath is passed over the dilator. The dilator is then removed and the endoscope is then inserted. Continuous irrigation with 0.9% saline is started. Local anatomy is then established.

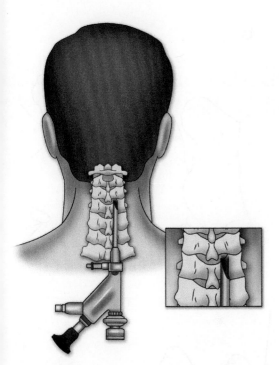

Fig. 1. Anteroposterior and lateral fluoroscopy is used to target the "Y" point with the endoscope. This "Y" is the lateral most point of the 2 lamina converging on the medial aspect of the facet joint. (Reprinted with permission, University of Wisconsin © 2019. All Rights Reserved.)

The target point of the outer working sheath is the "Y" point of the cranial lamina of the symptomatic side (see **Fig. 1**). This "Y" is the lateral most point of the 2 lamina converging on the medial aspect of the facet joint. Its boundaries are the inferior margin of the cranial lamina, the medial junction of the facet joints, and the superior margin of the caudal lamina. Residual muscle attached around the "Y" point is coagulated with the radiofrequency bipolar coagulator and removed. The interlaminar ligamentum flavum, inferior margin of the cranial lamina, superior margin of the caudal lamina, and medial aspect of the facet joint are exposed and visualized.

An endoscopic drill is used to begin the decompression from the lateral aspect of the cranial lamina extending laterally toward the apex of the interlaminar space and rostrally to the inferior articulating process.[20] In order to facilitate an appropriate field of view, tissue elasticity is used to provide a pivot point for the working cannula holding the endoscope and the drill for adequate visualization and for achieving sufficient bony decompression. This is the so called "joystick technique." The sequence of drilling is as follows (**Fig. 2**):

1. Drilling starts at the lateral aspect of the cranial lamina and gradually extends to the medial aspect of the inferior articulating process. A protected side cutting drill is usually used. The extent of bone drilling depends on the size and location of the foramen and is usually within a 3 to 4 mm radius around the Y point. The extent of bone removal can be assessed, by comparing it with the size of the drill. The rostral goal is to decompress to a point at or just beyond the tip of the superior articulating process. If need be, drilling further superiorly to the caudal border of the rostral pedicle will allow access to the superior aspect of the foramen. The lateral drilling can extend to the lateral border of the pedicle (the most lateral aspect of the foramen). Resection of more than 50% of the facet joint should be avoided to avoid instability.[21–23]

2. Next the superior articulating process (SAP) of the caudal vertebrae is thinned beginning at the rostral tip of the SAP and ending at the superior border of the caudal pedicle. Typically, a rough diamond burr is effective in thinning the bone and limiting the risk of dural injury. A micro-Kerrison ronguer is used to remove the thinned SAP.

3. The shoulder and/or the axilla of the nerve root is carefully explored if a free disc fragment needs to be removed. Typically, disc fragments will be located in the axilla of the exiting nerve root. Once the lateral edge of the thecal sac has been exposed, the open bevel of the working channel is kept directed medially, to avoid compression of the thecal sac. Care must also be taken to avoid iatrogenic injury to the nerve. The nerve root may be separated into dorsal and ventral bundles. During the posterior percutaneous endoscopic procedure Ruetten and colleagues[24] were able to see separate ventral and dorsal bundles in about 20% of cases. The end point of the procedure is the visualization of a freely mobile nerve root. Decompression may be confirmed at both the superior and inferior margin of the nerve root, by palpation with a blunt probe.

4. Hemostasis is established.

5. The skin is generally closed with a single absorbable stitch.

Additional tools and working sheaths can be used but are not typically used by the senior author. An outer working sheath with a longer bevel has also been recommended by some, as the bevel tip may be used to manipulate and retract roots without the risk of pressing on the thecal sac. A side-firing holmium:yttrium-aluminium-garnet or CO_2 laser[25] may be used through the working channel to extend soft tissue resection in the axilla and along the root laterally.

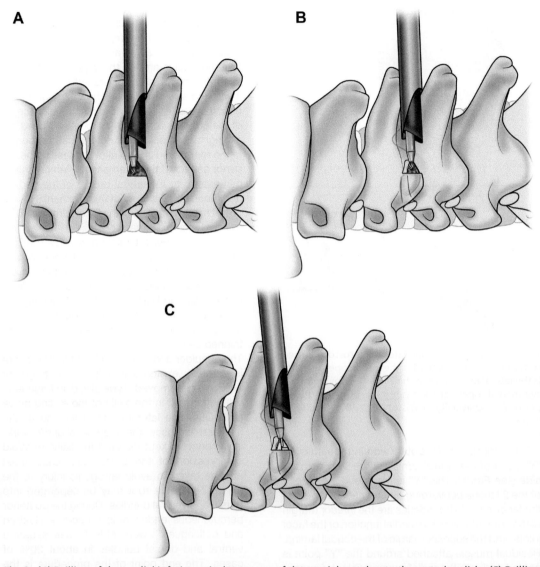

Fig. 2. (*A*) Drilling of the medial inferior articular process of the cranial vertebra to the rostral pedicle. (*B*) Drilling of the medial superior articular process of the inferior vertebra to the caudal pedicle. (*C*) Removal of the herniated disc from the axilla of the nerve root, if needed. Complete decompression can be verified by observing free floating neural structures and palpating with flexible probes. (Reprinted with permission, University of Wisconsin © 2019. All Rights Reserved.)

If a second or third level of foraminal pathology needs to be addressed, the instruments are removed, and using the same incision and tissue elasticity, under fluoroscopy, a dilator is redirected and placed through a new track at the medial facet joint to be addressed. The procedure is then repeated.

Outcomes and Complications

Endoscopic posterior cervical foraminotomy would be an attractive procedure if outcomes and complication profile were to be equivalent to other established procedures. The appeal of the endoscopic procedure lies in achieving a foraminotomy (and if needed excision of a laterally herniated disc fragment), with minimal approach-related trauma to the normal structures overlying the facet joint. This may be advantageous for the patient, leading to less postoperative incisional pain, less use of opioids, early return to work, and potentially less risk of postoperative infection.

A review of the literature to assess the outcomes and complication profile of posterior foraminotomies in general, and fully endoscopic posterior foraminotomies in particular, follows.

Anterior cervical discectomy and fusion versus open foraminotomy

Several studies have shown the equivalence of clinical outcomes and complication rates when comparing open foraminotomies and ACDF for unilateral lateral disc herniation and foraminal stenosis.[1,15,26] Cost-analysis studies however do favor posterior foraminotomy over anterior cervical discectomy and show significantly lower costs for the foraminotomy group.[5,6,27] Adverse events were noted to be more frequent and costs higher in the ACDF group as compared with the posterior cervical foraminotomy group.[6] Dohrmann and Hsieh[28] analyzed long-term results of 6000 patients comparing anterior versus posterior approaches and noted that the posterior approaches had significantly better outcomes. Two main concerns with posterior cervical foraminotomies have been the risk of index level segmental kyphosis and neck and shoulder pain thought to be from muscle stripping with the open procedure. A prevalence of neck pain 10% to 20% has been reported after open posterior foraminotomy procedures.[4,8,29] An increase in kyphosis or evidence of instability at the index or adjacent segment, following a posterior foraminotomy, has not been evident.[30]

Anterior cervical discectomy and fusion versus minimally invasive or endoscopic posterior foraminotomy

Studies assessing posterior cervical foraminotomies, either fully endoscopic or using a tubular access system, have reported good or excellent relief of pain, similar to outcomes of ACDF or open cervical foraminotomies.[4,8,9,31,32] Ruetten and colleagues[24] published a direct comparison of fully endoscopic posterior cervical foraminotomy to standard ACDF and did not find any significant differences in outcomes or complications. They also noted a reduced operating time (28 vs 68 minutes mean) and a faster return to work time (19 vs 34 days) with the endoscopic technique. Numerous other studies have also shown that anterior cervical discectomy and minimally invasive posterior cervical foraminotomy procedure have comparable outcomes.[4,10,33–36]

Open foraminotomy versus minimally invasive tubular access foraminotomy

A meta-analysis compared open foraminotomy with minimally invasive techniques, although only one of the included studies used a full-endoscopic technique. The investigators reported that the pooled clinical success rate was 92.7% for open procedures, as opposed to 94.9% for minimally invasive approaches.[37] Clark and colleagues[38] in a systematic review analyzed 19 publications and found that patients undergoing percutaneous cervical laminoforaminotomy have lower blood loss, a shorter surgical time, less inpatient analgesic use, and a shorter hospital stay compared with patients undergoing open procedures. Kim and colleagues[39] also found equivalent outcomes among the 2 groups.

Fully endoscopic posterior cervical foraminotomy for foraminal osseous stenosis

Ohmori and colleagues[40] compared patients with lateral disc herniation spondylotic foraminal stenosis. Both groups had similar facetectomy with an average of 52% of facet resection and no difference in outcomes. Other investigators have also shown good clinical outcomes and a low rate of complications in patients with foraminal osseous stenosis.[41]

Motion and posterior cervical foraminotomy

Cho and colleagues[42] have shown in a study of 31 patients who underwent posterior cervical foraminotomy that motion at the operated segment and adjacent segments was not significantly affected. In comparison, patients who underwent ACDF had significant decrease in motion at the operated segment and significant increase in motion at especially the caudal level. Jagannathan and colleagues[17] reviewed a series of 162 patients, who underwent posterior cervical radiculopathy, and noted that a loss of lordosis (segmental Cobb angle <10°) was seen in 18.5% of their patients in follow-up ranging from 60 to 177 months. In addition, age greater than 60 years was also a risk factor for worsening of sagittal alignment. However, Won and colleagues[16] in their series looked at this specific issue and noted that posterior endoscopic foraminotomy was effective in reducing radicular symptoms and that preexisting loss of cervical lordosis (segmental Cobb angle <10°) did not lead to worse outcomes, and no worsening of lordosis was apparent albeit with a shorter follow-up period.

Risk of reoperation at same level

The rate of same-level reoperation (6.6%) has been noted to be similar to reoperations after ACDF.[43] Minimally invasive posterior cervical foraminotomy for the treatment of cervical radiculopathy demonstrated rates of revision at index and adjacent levels no different than those following ACDF.[11] Wang and colleagues[44] report the rate of a subsequent anterior cervical fusion procedure following posterior cervical foraminotomy and note that the 5% rate of reoperation is similar to the historical rate of revision after ACDF. Skovrlj and colleagues[45] followed 70 patients who underwent minimally invasive tubular access posterior foraminotomies and found that there was a low rate (1.1% per index level per year) of future index site fusion. Lubelski and colleagues[46] similarly found that the reoperation rate at the index level was 4.8% for the ACDF group and 6.4% for the posterior cervical foraminotomy group (*P* = .7) within 2 years of the initial surgery.

Complications

Posterior endoscopic cervical foraminotomy is associated with few complications. In a single-center review of 249 cases, 3 cases had to be revised with ACDF and one patient required evacuation of an epidural hematoma. Dural injury occurred in one patient.[47] Similarly, Ruetten and colleagues,[12,32] in a randomized trial of ACDF compared with posterior cervical endoscopic foraminotomy/discectomy, noted few complications and similar outcomes.

A review of the literature suggests that both anterior and posterior techniques for cervical radiculopathy have similar outcomes. The complication profiles of anterior and posterior approaches are different as is to be expected from the different anatomic structures encountered, but the rates for both are low and similar. Posterior approaches in general and minimally invasive surgery or fully endoscopic techniques in particular enjoy the advantage of shorter procedure, shorter hospital stay, and early return to work with significantly lower costs associated with the procedure itself. As data accumulate over time, a more advantageous profile of a fully endoscopic technique may become apparent.

SUMMARY

For patients with unilateral cervical radiculopathy refractory to conservative management from lateral disc herniation or degenerative spondylotic foraminal stenosis, a posterior endoscopic cervical foraminotomy should be considered. The outcomes with this technique are equivalent to any other technique, approach-related tissue damage is minimized, and tissue preservation is maximized. This technique addresses the pathology directly and is cost-effective compared with the standard ACDF. Risks and complications have been minimal in several series. There may be a long learning curve for proficiency in endoscopic techniques. Familiarity with other endoscopic procedures may shorten the learning curve for this procedure.

SUPPLEMENTARY DATA

Supplementary data related to this article can be found online at https://doi.org/10.1016/j.nec.2019.08.001.

REFERENCES

1. Henderson Charles M, Hennessy Robert G, Shuey Henry M, et al. Posterior-lateral foraminotomy as an exclusive operative technique for cervical radiculopathy: a review of 846 consecutively operated cases. Neurosurgery 1983;13(5):504–12.
2. Krupp W, Schattke H, Müke R. Clinical results of the foraminotomy as described by Frykholm for the treatment of lateral cervical disc herniation. Acta Neurochir 1990;107(1–2):22–9.
3. Aldrich F. Posterolateral microdiscectomy for cervical monoradiculopathy caused by posterolateral soft cervical disc sequestration. J Neurosurg 1990;72(3):370–7.
4. Grieve JP, Kitchen ND, Moore AJ, et al. Results of posterior cervical foraminotomy for treatment of cervical spondylitic radiculopathy. Br J Neurosurg 2009;14(1):40–3.
5. Tumialán Luis M, Ponton Ryan P, Gluf Wayne M. Management of unilateral cervical radiculopathy in the military: the cost effectiveness of posterior cervical foraminotomy compared with anterior cervical discectomy and fusion. Neurosurg Focus 2010;28(5):E17.
6. Witiw CD, Smieliauskas F, O'Toole JE, et al. Comparison of anterior cervical discectomy and fusion to posterior cervical foraminotomy for cervical radiculopathy: utilization, costs, and adverse events 2003-2014. Neurosurgery 2018;5:1–8.
7. Kerry G, Hammer A, Ruedinger C, et al. Microsurgical posterior cervical foraminotomy: a study of 181 cases. Br J Neurosurg 2017;31(1):39–44.
8. Hilton DL Jr. Minimally invasive tubular access for posterior cervical foraminotomy with three-dimensional microscopic visualization and localization with anterior/posterior imaging. Spine J 2007;7(2):154–8.
9. Coric D, Adamson T. Minimally invasive cervical microendoscopic laminoforaminotomy. Neurosurg Focus 2008;25(2):E2.
10. Burke TG, Caputy A. Microendoscopic posterior cervical foraminotomy: a cadaveric model and clinical application for cervical radiculopathy. J Neurosurg 2000;93(1 Suppl):126–9.
11. Dunn C, Moore J, Sahai N, et al. Minimally invasive posterior cervical foraminotomy with tubes to prevent undesired fusion: a long-term follow-up study. J Neurosurg Spine 2018;93(1):358–64.
12. Ruetten S, Komp M, Merk H, et al. A new full-endoscopic technique for cervical posterior

foraminotomy in the treatment of lateral disc herniations using 6.9-mm endoscopes: prospective 2-year results of 87 patients. Minim Invasive Neurosurg 2007;50(04):219–26.

13. Gu BS, Park JH, Seong HY, et al. Feasibility of posterior cervical foraminotomy in cervical foraminal stenosis. Spine 2017;42(5):E267–71.

14. Young RM, Leiphart JW, Shields DC, et al. Anterior cervical fusion versus minimally invasive posterior keyhole decompression for cervical radiculopathy. Interdiscip Neurosurg 2015;2(4):169–76.

15. Liu WJ, Hu L, Chou PH, et al. Comparison of anterior cervical discectomy and fusion versus posterior cervical foraminotomy in the treatment of cervical radiculopathy: a systematic review. Orthop Surg 2016; 8(4):425–31.

16. Won S, Kim CH, Chung CK, et al. Clinical outcomes of single-level posterior percutaneous endoscopic cervical foraminotomy for patients with less cervical lordosis. J Minim Invasive Spine Surg Tech 2016; 1(1):11–7.

17. Jagannathan J, Sherman JH, Szabo T, et al. The posterior cervical foraminotomy in the treatment of cervical disc/osteophyte disease: a single-surgeon experience with a minimum of 5 years' clinical and radiographic follow-up. J Neurosurg Spine 2009; 73(1):347–56.

18. Czervionke LF, Daniels DL, Ho PS, et al. Cervical neural foramina: correlative anatomic and MR imaging study. Radiology 1988;169(3):753–9.

19. Daniels DL, Grogan JP, Johansen JG, et al. Cervical radiculopathy: computed tomography and myelography compared. Radiology 1984;151(1):109–13.

20. Kravtsov MN, Liulin SV, Kuznetsov MV, et al. Fully endoscopic posterior cervical foraminotomy and discectomy for lateral disc herhiation (literature review and results of authors' studies). Genij Ortopedii 2018;24(2):240–51.

21. Raynor RB. Anterior or posterior approach to the cervical spine: an anatomical and radiographic evaluation and comparison. Neurosurgery 1983;12(1): 7–13.

22. Zdeblick TA, Zou D, Warden KE, et al. Cervical stability after foraminotomy. A biomechanical in vitro analysis. J Bone Joint Surg Am 1992;74(1):22–7.

23. Zdeblick TA, Abitbol JJ, Kunz DN, et al. Cervical stability after sequential capsule resection. Spine 1993; 18(14):2005–8.

24. Ruetten S, Komp M, Merk H, et al. Full-endoscopic cervical posterior foraminotomy for the operation of lateral disc herniations using 5.9-mm endoscopes: a prospective, randomized, controlled study. Spine 2008;33(9):940–8.

25. Jeon HC, Kim CS, Kim SC, et al. Posterior cervical microscopic foraminotomy and discectomy with laser for unilateral radiculopathy. Chonnam Med J 2015;51(3):129–34.

26. Selvanathan SK, Beagrie C, Thomson S, et al. Anterior cervical discectomy and fusion versus posterior cervical foraminotomy in the treatment of brachialgia: the Leeds spinal unit experience (2008–2013). Acta Neurochir 2015;157(9):1595–600.

27. Mansfield HE. Single-level anterior cervical discectomy and fusion versus minimally invasive posterior cervical foraminotomy for patients with cervical radiculopathy: a cost analysis. Neurosurg Focus 2014; 1–5. https://doi.org/10.3171/2014.8.FOCUS14373.

28. Dohrmann GJ, Hsieh JC. Long-term results of anterior versus posterior operations for herniated cervical discs: analysis of 6,000 patients. Med Princ Pract 2014;23(1):70–3.

29. Clarke MJ, Ecker RD, Krauss WE, et al. Same-segment and adjacent-segment disease following posterior cervical foraminotomy. J Neurosurg Spine 2007;6(1):5–9.

30. Kwon YJ. Long-term clinical and radiologic outcomes of minimally invasive posterior cervical foraminotomy. J Korean Neurosurg Soc 2014;56(3): 224–6.

31. O'Toole JE, Sheikh H, Eichholz KM, et al. Endoscopic posterior cervical foraminotomy and discectomy. Neurosurg Clin N Am 2006;17(4): 411–22.

32. Ruetten S, Komp M, Merk H, et al. Full-endoscopic anterior decompression versus conventional anterior decompression and fusion in cervical disc herniations. Int Orthop 2008;33(6):1677–82.

33. Woertgen C, Rothoerl RD, Henkel J, et al. Long term outcome after cervical foraminotomy. J Clin Neurosci 2000;7(4):312–5.

34. Laing RJ, Ng I, Seeley HM, et al. Prospective study of clinical and radiological outcome after anterior cervical discectomy. Br J Neurosurg 2001;15(4): 319–23.

35. Sonntag VK, Han PP, Vishteh AG. Anterior cervical discectomy. Neurosurgery 2001;49(4):909–12.

36. Cağlar YS, Bozkurt M, Kahilogullari G, et al. Keyhole approach for posterior cervical discectomy: experience on 84 patients. Minim Invasive Neurosurg 2007;50(1):7–11.

37. McAnany SJ, Kim JS, Overley SC, et al. A meta-analysis of cervical foraminotomy: open versus minimally-invasive techniques. Spine J 2015;15(5): 849–56.

38. Clark JG, Abdullah KG, Steinmetz MP, et al. Minimally invasive versus open cervical foraminotomy: a systematic review. Global Spine J 2011;1(1): 009–14.

39. Kim CH, Kim KT, Chung CK, et al. Minimally invasive cervical foraminotomy and diskectomy for laterally located soft disk herniation. Eur Spine J 2015; 24(12):3005–12.

40. Ohmori K, Ono K, Hori T. Outcomes of full-endoscopic posterior cervical foraminotomy for

cervical radiculopathy caused by bony stenosis of the intervertebral foramen. Mini-invasive Surg 2017;1(2):1–6.

41. Oertel JM, Philipps M, Burkhardt BW. Endoscopic posterior cervical foraminotomy as a treatment for osseous foraminal stenosis. World Neurosurg 2016;91(C):50–7.

42. Cho TG, Kim YB, Park SW. Long term effect on adjacent segment motion after posterior cervical foraminotomy. Korean J Spine 2014;11(1):1–6.

43. Bydon M, Mathios D, Macki M. Long-term patient outcomes after posterior cervical foraminotomy: an analysis of 151 cases. J Neurosurg Spine 2014;21:727–31.

44. Wang TY, Lubelski D, Abdullah KG, et al. Rates of anterior cervical discectomy and fusion after initial posterior cervical foraminotomy. Spine J 2015; 15(5):971–6.

45. Skovrlj B, Gologorsky Y, Haque R, et al. Complications, outcomes, and need for fusion after minimally invasive posterior cervical foraminotomy and microdiscectomy. Spine J 2014;14(10):2405–11.

46. Lubelski D, Healy AT, Silverstein MP, et al. Reoperation rates after anterior cervical discectomy and fusion versus posterior cervical foraminotomy: a propensity-matched analysis. Spine J 2015;15(6): 1277–83.

47. Zheng C, Huang X, Yu J, et al. Posterior percutaneous endoscopic cervical diskectomy: a single-center experience of 252 cases. World Neurosurg 2018;120:e63–7.

Endoscopic Lumbar Interbody Fusion

G. Damian Brusko, BS[a],*, Michael Y. Wang, MD[b]

KEYWORDS

- Endoscopic • Lumbar fusion • Interbody fusion • Minimally invasive • Enhanced recovery

KEY POINTS

- The indications for endoscopic lumbar interbody fusion (LIF) are similar to those of standard TLIF procedures: lumbar degenerative pathologies and low-grade spondylolisthesis.
- The techniques for endoscopic LIF have evolved over time, transitioning from modifications of the tubular retractor approach to awake uniportal endoscopic fusion.
- Endoscopic LIF may play a future role in enhanced recovery programs as reductions in pain and length of hospital result in faster postoperative recovery for patients with lasting clinical improvements.
- Both minor and major complications can result from endoscopic spine surgery, particularly in inexperienced hands.

INTRODUCTION

Spine surgery is continuously evolving, yet the goal of surgery remains the same: maximize outcomes and minimize morbidity. Over many decades, spine surgeons have adopted several surgical techniques, technologies, and treatments to achieve this goal. Advances in minimally invasive surgery (MIS) have afforded the opportunity for increased access to spine procedures for elderly and comorbid patients who are at increased risk of morbidity with traditional open spine surgery. As the elderly population continues to grow and rates of spine surgery increase, MIS techniques will likely have an even greater impact. Thus, spine surgeons have recently developed more advanced and less invasive techniques. One significant example of recent surgical innovation is the advent of endoscopic-assisted spine surgery. Applications of the endoscope are prevalent in a variety of procedures from the cervical to lumbar spine. This review focuses specifically on endoscopic lumbar interbody fusion (LIF) and details the specific indications, techniques, outcomes, and complications associated with these procedures.

INDICATIONS

As with any surgical procedure, careful patient selection should be exercised when choosing a surgical approach. A benefit of endoscopic LIF surgeries is that they may be a preferable alternative for patients unable to tolerate open lumbar fusion. Those at risk of complications, particularly the elderly, or patients desiring the least morbid or most cosmetically acceptable surgical option would likely benefit from endoscopic LIF. A

Financial Disclosures: G.D. Brusko: None. M.Y. Wang: royalty payments from DePuy-Synthes Spine, Inc, Children's Hospital of Los Angeles, Springer Publishing, and Quality Medical Publishing; consultant for DePuy-Synthes Spine, Inc, Stryker Spine, K2M, and Spineology; advisory board member for Vallum; stock in Spinicity and Innovative Surgical Devices; and grants from the Department of Defense.

[a] Department of Neurological Surgery, University of Miami Miller School of Medicine, Lois Pope Life Center, 1095 Northwest 14th Terrace, Miami, FL 33136, USA; [b] Department of Neurological Surgery, University of Miami Miller School of Medicine, 1095 Northwest 14th Terrace, Miami, FL 33136, USA
* Corresponding author.
E-mail address: g.brusko@med.miami.edu

combination of shorter operative times, reduced pain, and smaller incisions make endoscopic lumbar fusion appealing to such patients.

Clinical indications for endoscopic LIF are evolving, but are generally the same as those for traditional minimally invasive interbody fusions: degenerative lumbar pathologies (including disk herniation, spinal stenosis with instability, and mild-moderate central stenosis with concomitant foraminal stenosis) and low-grade (Meyerding grade I-II) spondylolisthesis (**Table 1**).[1] Early experiences with one- and two-level endoscopic fusions were most common, but as techniques improve, multilevel fusions will likely also be attempted.

Patients with severe bilateral and central canal stenosis may benefit more from a biportal endoscopic technique, which enables better access to the contralateral side than a uniportal approach through Kambin triangle. Other contraindications to interbody fusion include patients with osteoporotic bone, which impedes indirect compression because pressure on the end plates is required to lift the intervertebral space,[2] and patients with bilateral radiculopathy in whom unilateral neural decompression may not adequately relieve symptoms.[3]

Indications for endoscopic LIF are similar to those of standard transforaminal LIF (TLIF) procedures, but may be offered to nontraditional spine surgery patients, including the elderly or those with multiple comorbidities. As experience with endoscopic fusion techniques increases, many surgeons may expand the range of clinical indications for these minimally invasive procedures.

TECHNIQUE

Surgical techniques for using endoscopes in lumbar fusion have evolved since their inception more than a decade ago. The most common and well-described procedure is the TLIF, but more recent studies have begun to detail endoscopic lateral LIF (LLIF). Each of these techniques is discussed separately in this section.

Endoscopic Transforaminal Lumbar Interbody Fusion

Introduction of the endoscope-assisted TLIF occurred in 2008; an endoscope was inserted into a tubular retractor to aid in decompression and discectomy.[4] This combination of tubular retractor and endoscope has been described in other studies with select modifications: use of a narrow-surface fusion cage[5] and intraoperative computer navigation assistance with cone-beam computed tomography.[6] However, reliance on the tubular retractor for access to the interbody space and the endoscope for visualization did not constitute a fully endoscopic approach.

Subsequently, surgeons developed other techniques for endoscopic TLIF, such as the biportal endoscopic approach. Similar to MIS-TLIF using tubular retractors, removal of bony structures is required.[7,8] Heo and colleagues[8] describe their unilateral biportal endoscopic technique for TLIF. Two paramedian skin incisions are made above and below the midportion of the spinous process or disk space and the ipsilateral medial border of the pedicle. Serial dilation of the skin incisions is completed to create two channels: one working and one endoscopic channel. The ipsilateral lamina is then removed, and neural decompression is achieved with complete visualization of the nerve roots aided by the endoscopic channel. Ipsilateral facetectomy is completed next, followed by discectomy and cartilaginous end plate removal. Autograft and a long, straight interbody cage are placed deep into the intervertebral space. Ipsilateral percutaneous pedicle screws are inserted through the same skin incisions and an additional two skin incisions are made contralaterally for the other pair of pedicle screws.

As endoscopic TLIF procedures and technologies evolved, a transition to even more minimally invasive techniques took place, which minimized muscular dissection even further with a single, smaller channel and obviated unilateral facetectomy. Our institution's first report in the literature from 2016 describes the initial series of 10 patients who underwent an ultraminimally invasive endoscopic TLIF without the use of general anesthesia.[2] Importantly, using sedation rather than

Table 1	
Indications for endoscopic lumbar interbody fusion	
Indications	Relative Contraindications/ Considerations
Degenerative disk disease	Severe bilateral stenosis
Spinal stenosis with instability	Severe central stenosis
Mild-moderate central stenosis with concomitant unilateral foraminal stenosis	Patients with osteoporosis
Low-grade spondylolisthesis (grade I-II)	Patients with bilateral radiculopathy

general anesthesia allows for enhanced live feedback from the patient to the surgeon related to proximity of neural elements during decompression. The technique consists of a series of critical steps outlined in **Table 2** and is summarized here.

Following positioning of the patient prone on a Jackson table, needle localization of the lumbar disk space under simultaneous anteroposterior and lateral fluoroscopy is completed. Successive dilation is performed to create an 8-mm working channel, which is small enough to allow room for the endoscopic working channel and exiting nerve root. The endoscope is placed through the channel and the nerve roots are visualized before decompression (**Fig. 1**), which involves a combination of bipolar cautery, pituitary rongeurs, osteotomes, curettes, and powered drills. Use of the endoscope allows direct visualization to achieve adequate decompression, followed by discectomy and end plate preparation. One technical refinement made after the initial series of patients was the use of an inflatable balloon within the disk space that is filled with radiopaque contrast to determine if sufficient cartilaginous end plate was removed.[9] Next, recombinant human bone morphogenic protein is placed in the anterior

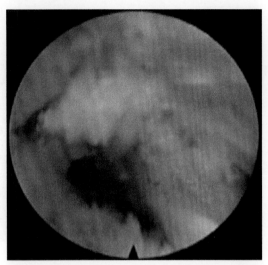

Fig. 1. Image from an endoscopic video during endoscopic TLIF illustrating decompression of the nerve root in the foramen.

disk space and visualized with a small amount of iohexol on fluoroscopy to ensure proper placement. An expandable mesh interbody cage is then placed in the interbody space and packed with allograft until disk height restoration and reduction of any spondylolisthesis has been achieved (**Fig. 2**). The working channel is removed, and percutaneous pedicle screw fixation is performed to complete to interbody fusion.

Important to note is the critical step of localizing of the disk space. Knowledge of Kambin's triangle, which allows transforaminal access to several structures, including the traversing and exiting nerve roots, thecal sac, and disk space, is crucial to obtain proper access for endoscopic portion of the case. Kambin first described his technique for percutaneous discectomy that involved obliquely entering the disk space through a triangle, the borders of which are made up of the exiting nerve root anteriorly, the traversing root medially, and the lateral aspect of the superior articular process of the inferior vertebral segment posteriorly (**Fig. 3**).[10] Kambin's technique precludes the need for a complete facetectomy to achieve adequate visualization of the traversing root because of the 35° angle into the neural foramen. In contrast, Harms' technique for TLIF that uses this triangle describes a 15° to 20° angle, which mandates a facetectomy for proper visualization.[11] Disagreements regarding these two approaches to Kambin's triangle for endoscopic TLIF have been discussed, with recent proponents suggesting the original triangle should be described in three dimensions as "Kambin's prism" (**Fig. 4**).[12]

Table 2
Surgical technique for the endoscopic transforaminal lumbar interbody fusion

	Procedural Step
1	Patient positioned prone on Jackson table
2	Needle localization of disk space via Kambin's triangle
3	Successive dilation of incision to create 8-mm working channel
4	Endoscopic-assisted nerve root decompression
5	Endoscopic-assisted discectomy and end plate preparation
6	Recombinant human bone morphogenic protein followed by interbody cage placement in disk space
7	Filling of expandable interbody cage with bone graft
8	Removal of working channel
9	Placement of percutaneous pedicle screws
10	Insertion of rods percutaneously to connect pedicle screws
11	Figure-of-eight sutures to close each small incision

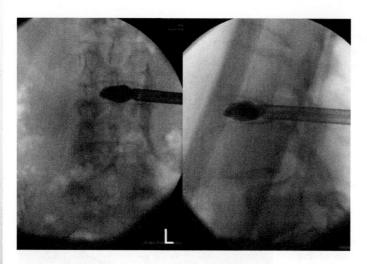

Fig. 2. Anteroposterior (*left*) and lateral (*right*) intraoperative fluoroscopy images of the expandable interbody cage filled with allograft to achieve adequate indirect decompression of the nerve root.

Endoscopic Lateral Lumbar Interbody Fusions

Although literature on endoscopic TLIF has grown tremendously in the last several years, only two articles describe techniques for endoscopic LLIF procedures. Schonauer and colleagues[13] describe the first use of an endoscope-assisted extreme LLIF (EA-XLIF). The endoscope assists in visualization of the course of the genitofemoral nerve and disk surface before shim and retractor placement. The discectomy is completed under direct visualization via the endoscope, which is then inserted into the interbody space to verify end plate integrity, orientation, and contralateral annulus release. The endoscope is again used to confirm proper cage placement, and on removal

of the self-retaining retractor, it is used to ensure adequate hemostasis and psoas reassembly has been achieved.

Kyoh[14] recently published a series of patients who underwent endoscopic LLIF, attempting to mitigate potential complications associated with more-invasive LLIF procedures. An original endoscopic spine surgery system and a series of dilators were developed to facilitate the technique. A single 2-cm skin incision is made at the anterior border of the vertebral body at the appropriate level. Muscular dissection and placement of the endoscopic working channel in the retroperitoneum through intermuscular crevice is completed, which aids in visualization of structures. An initial long dilator is used to traverse the psoas muscle

Fig. 3. Illustrative graphic of Kambin's triangle used to safely access the disk space during an endoscopic TLIF.

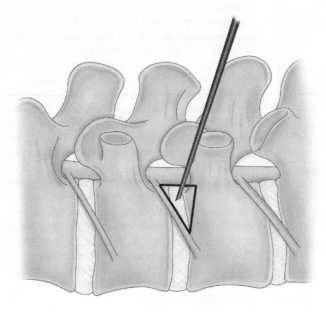

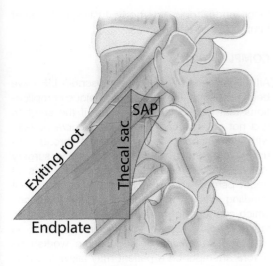

Fig. 4. Illustrative graphic of the newly proposed Kambin's prism approach for endoscopic TLIF. SAP, superior articular process.

and allows for tactile feedback once the protruding disk is reached. Additional dilators and sheaths serve as different-sized channels for various instruments used during the discectomy, end plate preparation, and cage insertion.

Techniques for endoscopic TLIF have transitioned from reliance on tubular retractors for access to uniportal approaches that maximally reduce the amount of tissue disruption required. In-depth knowledge of Kambin's triangle (or prism) is essential to properly access the interbody space if facetectomy is to be avoided. Although reports of endoscopic LLIF are limited at present, it is likely that surgeons will soon adapt new techniques and technologies to further develop this approach.

OUTCOMES

The development and improvement of endoscopic LIF techniques described has resulted in a substantial benefit for patients in several aspects. Although clinical outcomes, such as acute pain reduction and faster postoperative recovery, are the primary drivers for adoption of minimally invasive endoscopic techniques, improvements in radiographic outcomes, long-term patient-reported outcome measures (PROMs), and hospitalization costs have also been well-described.

One example of the multifaceted impact of endoscopic lumbar surgery is our previously described awake endoscopic TLIF.[2] The average age of the initial 10 patients in this series was 62.2 years with the oldest patient aged 78 years. Patients experienced minimal blood loss and reduced operative times of less than 2 hours on

average, leading to a mean length of hospital stay (LOS) of just 1.4 days. At 1-year follow-up, none of the initial 10 patients demonstrated radiographic nonunion on imaging. Importantly, the clinical benefits in patients were durable, with substantial improvements in 1-year Oswestry Disability Index (ODI), Short-Form Health Survey-36, and EQ-5D scores compared with preoperative baseline. In a follow-up study on the first 100 patients to undergo the awake endoscopic TLIF, reductions in blood loss, Operating Room (OR) time, and LOS were again seen.[9] A significant improvement in mean ODI difference from baseline to 1-year follow-up of −12.3 points was observed for this group of 100 patients.

Other programs have demonstrated similar outcomes using the biportal endoscopic technique. The average patient age ranged from 68.7 years (oldest patient aged 85 years) to 71.2 years, demonstrating that many spine surgeons are choosing endoscopic approaches as a viable option for lumbar fusion in this patient population.[7,8] Although operative times are longer for this technique (mean, 165–169 min), blood loss remained less than 100 mL and significant postoperative improvements in Visual Analog Scale (VAS) and ODI were observed at 2 months and 1 year follow-up periods.[7,8] Similarly at 1-year follow-up, patients undergoing early endoscopic TLIFs through a tubular retractor demonstrated improvements clinically on VAS, ODI, and Japanese Orthopedic Association scores, and radiographically, with all 17 patients achieving solid bone graft fusion during this time period.[6]

Yang and colleagues,[15] randomized a series of 100 patients to undergo either microendoscopic-assisted MIS-TLIF or open TLIF. The MIS group was associated with significantly less blood loss and postoperative nonsteroidal anti-inflammatory drug use, ambulation 2 days earlier, and sustained improvements in ODI, VAS, and Japanese Orthopedic Association scores at 1-month and 2-year follow-up compared with the open TLIF group. Interbody fusion rate was similar between groups (88% MIS vs 90% open). However, in contrast to other endoscopic fusion studies, mean surgical duration was significantly longer in the MIS group (178 minutes) compared with the open group (146 minutes) for single-level TLIF, as was intraoperative fluoroscopic time. Long-term results from this patient series reported comparable PROM scores between the MIS and open cohorts 5 years postoperatively.[16] This suggests that although endoscopic TLIF provides early clinical benefits compared with more invasive procedures, the long-term impact seems similar.

Furthermore, reducing the morbidities of the acute postoperative period allows for a greater impact on LOS and cost, which may factor into a health care system's initiative to develop an endoscopic spine surgery program. Much like the aims of endoscopic LIF, Enhanced Recovery After Surgery (ERAS) programs serve to limit pain, reduce complications, and decrease LOS through a multimodal, perioperative pathway.[17] Endoscopic TLIF as a central component of an ERAS pathway for lumbar fusion, in addition to conscious sedation and liposomal bupivacaine, has proven to be successful in significantly reducing pain, narcotic consumption, and LOS.[18,19] Additionally, this program resulted in significant acute care cost savings of $3444 (15.2% reduction) compared with a standard MIS-TLIF, which resulted primarily from shorter OR time and intensive care unit stays.[20] Application of ERAS with other endoscopic, nonawake fusion techniques has also demonstrated similar benefits in the acute recovery period.[21] The feasibility of fully endoscopic TLIF in an ambulatory surgery center has also been examined. A retrospective review of a 4-year experience concluded that fully endoscopic TLIF was a safe outpatient procedure for various patient populations, including the obese and elderly.[22] Therefore, the true value and future utility of endoscopic LIF may be as a central component of ERAS programs or in ambulatory surgery centers.

Additionally, for patients who underwent endoscopic LLIF, OR time decreased to 82.6 minutes during the last 20 patients in the series with little to no blood loss in any case and a reduction in average Numeric Rating Scale (NRS) score from 7.0 to 1.4 was observed.[14] Significant restoration in disk and foraminal heights and increased lumbar lordosis were also achieved. Patients who underwent the EA-XLIF experienced improvements in clinical outcomes at 6 weeks postoperatively.[13]

Outcomes for endoscopic LIF seem to have the greatest impact on outcomes in the early postoperative period, such that reduced tissue disruption, blood loss, and operative time promote decreased pain, accelerate early ambulation, and facilitate shorter LOS. This results in an overall improvement in PROMs. Importantly, these improvements are durable, because patients continue to report reduced pain compared with baseline at 1, 2, and 5 years postoperatively, even though differences in clinical and radiographic outcomes seem to equilibrate during long-term follow-up. However, when taken together, the benefits of enhanced postoperative recovery and stable long-term outcomes seem to favor endoscopic interbody fusion over other lumbar fusion approaches.

COMPLICATIONS

Although many benefits to endoscopic LIF have been examined, there are many unique complications that may occur, particularly if the surgeon has not yet reached the learning curve plateau with endoscopic cases. Several broad but unique challenges to endoscopic spine surgery include difficulty achieving hemostasis, loss of depth perception, disorientation, and instrument handling difficulty in the narrow working channel, which can lead to more serious complications in inexperienced hands.[23] Sufficient practice in cadaver laboratories or endoscopic workshops before attempts on a patient may alleviate many early difficulties.

The most commonly occurring minor complications include symptomatic epidural hematoma[8,21] and transient nerve root paraesthesias.[6] Other complications including dural tears,[7,8,16] L5 nerve root palsy,[7] muscle weakness caused by nerve retraction,[5] and medial pedicle screw breach of the central canal[5] and intraspinal hematoma[16] each requiring revision surgery have also been reported (**Table 3**). One initial study reported no complications in the first 10 patients.[2] After the first 100 patients, two cases of cage migration, one case of osteomyelitis, and one case of end plate fracture were identified, although three of these complications occurred during the surgeon's first 50 cases and technical refinements were subsequently implemented.[9] Additional studies have reported select cases of cage subsidence[21] and adjacent segment disease.[15]

Conversion from the awake anesthesia protocol to general anesthesia intraoperatively occurred successfully in all 4 patients of the initial 100 undergoing the awake endoscopic TLIF.[9] Two patients experienced emesis, one suffered epistaxis, and the final patient experienced extreme anxiety. However, no complications resulted from these

Table 3	
Common major and minor complications for endoscopic lumbar interbody fusion	
Major	**Minor**
Nerve root palsy	Epidural hematoma
Pedicle screw breach of spinal canal	Transient nerve root paraesthesias
Intraspinal hematoma	Dural tear
Cage migration	Transient psoas weakness (LLIF)

conversions, and the anesthetic protocol was modified to include improved antiemetic and epistaxis prophylaxis.

Although major complications of vascular injury and bowel perforation were avoided with the endoscopic LLIF, many of the common complications associated with traditional LLIF[24] were observed including transient psoas weakness, sensory disturbance of the thigh, and retroperitoneal injury with one resulting in postoperative ileus.[14] Four cases of cage migration requiring placement of a new cage were also demonstrated, for which additional technical refinements must be made. No patients suffered intraoperative complications during the EA-XLIF procedure, and just one experienced transient sensory thigh disturbance postoperatively.[13]

Overall, the incidences of intraoperative and postoperative complications with endoscopic TLIF seem to be minimal. Dural tears and transient nerve root palsy or muscle weakness may occur in more-invasive procedures, but unique challenges with the endoscope should warrant more careful consideration of such complications for surgeons. Additionally, several major neurologic and hardware complications resulted. Thus, surgeons should exercise caution and careful patient selection during the initial course of their learning curve with endoscopic LIF procedures to help mitigate the risk for more serious complications.

SUMMARY

Endoscopic LIF surgery was developed to further reduce the morbidity associated with more invasive lumbar fusion surgeries. The indications for endoscopic procedures are similar to those of traditional TLIF or LLIF procedures, including degenerative lumbar disease and low-grade spondylolisthesis and may also be the preferred options for select patients, such as the elderly. Techniques for endoscopic LIF have evolved over the past decade, progressively becoming even less invasive. During this transition to ultraminimally invasive endoscopic procedures, clinical and radiologic outcomes have improved, with particular benefits seen within ERAS pathways. However, as with any new surgical technology and technique, spine surgeons should be aware of the learning curve necessary before achieving operative mastery to minimize unique complications that can occur.

REFERENCES

1. Mobbs RJ, Phan K, Malham G, et al. Lumbar interbody fusion: techniques, indications and comparison of interbody fusion options including PLIF, TLIF, MI-TLIF, OLIF/ATP, LLIF and ALIF. J Spine Surg 2015;1(1):2–18.

2. Wang MY, Grossman J. Endoscopic minimally invasive transforaminal interbody fusion without general anesthesia: initial clinical experience with 1-year follow-up. Neurosurg Focus 2016;40(2):E13.

3. Foley KT, Holly LT, Schwender JD. Minimally invasive lumbar fusion. Spine 2003;28(15 Suppl):S26–35.

4. Zhou Y, Zhang C, Wang J, et al. Endoscopic transforaminal lumbar decompression, interbody fusion and pedicle screw fixation-a report of 42 cases. Chin J Traumatol 2008;11(4):225–31.

5. He EX, Guo J, Ling QJ, et al. Application of a narrow-surface cage in full endoscopic minimally invasive transforaminal lumbar interbody fusion. Int J Surg 2017;42:83–9.

6. Zhang Y, Xu C, Zhou Y, et al. Minimally invasive computer navigation-assisted endoscopic transforaminal interbody fusion with bilateral decompression via a unilateral approach: initial clinical experience at one-year follow-up. World Neurosurg 2017;106: 291–9.

7. Kim JE, Choi DJ. Biportal endoscopic transforaminal lumbar interbody fusion with arthroscopy. Clin Orthop Surg 2018;10(2):248–52.

8. Heo DH, Son SK, Eum JH, et al. Fully endoscopic lumbar interbody fusion using a percutaneous unilateral biportal endoscopic technique: technical note and preliminary clinical results. Neurosurg Focus 2017;43(2):E8.

9. Kolcun JPG, Brusko GD, Basil GW, et al. Endoscopic transforaminal lumbar interbody fusion without general anesthesia: operative and clinical outcomes in 100 consecutive patients with a minimum 1-year follow-up. Neurosurg Focus 2019; 46(4):E14.

10. Kambin P, Gellman H. Percutaneous lateral discectomy of the lumbar spine a preliminary report. Clin Orthop Relat Res 1983;174:127–32.

11. Harms JG, Jeszenszky D. Die posteriory lumbale, interkorporelle Fusion in unilateraler transforaminaler Technik. Oper Orthop Traumatol 1998; 10(2):90–102.

12. Tumialan LM, Madhavan K, Godzik J, et al. The history of and controversy over Kambin's triangle: a historical analysis of the lumbar transforaminal corridor for endoscopic and surgical approaches. World Neurosurg 2019;123:402–8.

13. Schonauer C, Stienen MN, Gautschi OP, et al. Endoscope-assisted extreme-lateral interbody fusion: preliminary experience and technical note. World Neurosurg 2017;103:869–75.e3.

14. Kyoh Y. Minimally invasive endoscopic-assisted lateral lumbar interbody fusion: technical report and preliminary results. Neurospine 2019;16(1): 72–81.

15. Yang Y, Liu B, Rong L-M, et al. Microendoscopy-assisted minimally invasive transforaminal lumbar interbody fusion for lumbar degenerative disease: short-term and medium-term outcomes. Int J Clin Exp Med 2015;8(11):21319–26.

16. Yang Y, Liu ZY, Zhang LM, et al. Microendoscopy-assisted minimally invasive versus open transforaminal lumbar interbody fusion for lumbar degenerative diseases: 5-year outcomes. World Neurosurg 2018; 116:e602–10.

17. Kehlet H. Multimodal approach to control postoperative pathophysiology and rehabilitation. Br J Anaesth 1997;78(5):606–17.

18. Wang MY, Chang PY, Grossman J. Development of an Enhanced Recovery After Surgery (ERAS) approach for lumbar spinal fusion. J Neurosurg Spine 2017;26(4):411–8.

19. Brusko GD, Kolcun JPG, Heger JA, et al. Reductions in length of stay, narcotics use, and pain following implementation of an enhanced recovery after surgery program for 1- to 3-level lumbar fusion surgery. Neurosurg Focus 2019; 46(4):E4.

20. Wang MY, Chang HK, Grossman J. Reduced acute care costs with the ERAS(R) minimally invasive transforaminal lumbar interbody fusion compared with conventional minimally invasive transforaminal lumbar interbody fusion. Neurosurgery 2018;83(4): 827–34.

21. Heo DH, Park CK. Clinical results of percutaneous biportal endoscopic lumbar interbody fusion with application of enhanced recovery after surgery. Neurosurg Focus 2019;46(4):E18.

22. Kamson S, Lu D, Sampson PD, et al. Full-endoscopic lumbar fusion outcomes in patients with minimal deformities: a retrospective study of data collected between 2011 and 2015. Pain Physician 2019;22(1):75–88.

23. Yadav YR, Lucano A, Ratre S, et al. Practical aspects and avoidance of complications in microendoscopic spine surgeries: a review. J Neurol Surg A Cent Eur Neurosurg 2019;80(4):291–301.

24. Cummock MD, Vanni S, Levi AD, et al. An analysis of postoperative thigh symptoms after minimally invasive transpsoas lumbar interbody fusion. J Neurosurg Spine 2011;15(1):11–8.

Endoscopic Lumbar Decompression

Sebastian Ruetten, MD*, Martin Komp, MD

KEYWORDS

- Degenerative lumbar spinal stenosis • Central spinal stenosis • Lateral spinal stenosis
- Spinal decompression • Full-endoscopic interlaminar approach
- Full-endoscopic transforaminal approach

KEY POINTS

- Full-endoscopic decompression of lumbar spinal canal stenosis is indicated if there are radicular symptoms in the legs and/or neurogenic claudication.
- Full-endoscopic decompression achieves good clinical results, has advantages, and can be performed as an alternative to standard procedures.
- The various full-endoscopic surgical approaches have individual indications and limitations.
- Full-endoscopic decompression operations can have a difficult learning curve.
- Conventional open and microsurgical methods may still need to be performed in order to react adequately to possible complications.

INTRODUCTION

Lumbar spinal canal stenoses usually manifest with radicular symptoms or neurogenic claudication. Back pain is more likely to be due to secondary degenerative phenomena. After exhausting conservative treatment options, if there is intolerable pain or neurologic deficits, a surgical procedure may be necessary. In this case, depending on the pathologic condition and symptoms, decompression surgery with or without fusion must be considered.[1,2] The overall trend is to move toward more selective, focused procedures. The current tendency for the lumbar spine is to perform a decompressive operation without fusion if there is not clear indication of segmental instability and the decompression will preserve stability.

Conventional decompression of the spine has good outcomes.[3] Nevertheless, approach-related, operation-specific problems and sequelae can occur that can negatively affect the results.[4] Therefore, from the very start of spinal surgery, attempts have been made to modify existing surgical techniques. The primary aim is to minimize trauma and its negative long-term effects and improve the surgical techniques, for example, by optimizing intraoperative visibility and light conditions. In this respect, the use of the microsurgical, microscope-assisted technique was a significant advance that is still established today.[5]

In general, more minimally invasive techniques can reduce tissue damage and its consequences.[6] Successful examples are endoscopic and endoscope-assisted operations that have become established in various fields of medicine. In the musculoskeletal system, arthroscopic operations under continuous irrigation have the advantages of being less invasive and enabling better intraoperative visibility.

Disclosure Statement: The authors have nothing to disclose.
Center for Spine Surgery and Pain Therapy, Center for Orthopaedics and Traumatology of the St. Elisabeth Group–Catholic Hospitals Rhein-Ruhr, St. Anna Hospital Herne/Marien Hospital Herne University Hospital/Marien Hospital Witten, Hospitalstr. 19, Herne 44649, Germany
* Corresponding author.
E-mail address: info@s-ruetten.com

The full-endoscopic technique is distinguished from endoscope-assisted transtubular approaches or other percutaneous, sometimes intradiscal methods.[7] This surgical technique of the spinal canal and adjacent structures under continuous view and irrigation is similar to an arthroscopy, but is a uniportal procedure using an endoscope with an intraendoscopic working channel. Endoscopes and instruments are available from various manufacturers. Rod lenses with a diameter of 6 to 7 mm and a view angle of around 25° that have an eccentric intraendoscopic working channel of around 4 mm are usually used today. The endoscope is inserted freely through a working sheath that retracts and protects surrounding tissue.

For a long time, the most common full-endoscopic technique on the lumbar spine was the posterolateral transforaminal approach.[8,9] In this technique, the spinal joints can obstruct direct access to the epidural space. The full-endoscopic lateral transforaminal approach was therefore developed with an approach trajectory 10° to 15° from the coronal plane, in which the spinal canal can be accessed directly under continuous view.[7,10] Nevertheless, intraspinal pathologic conditions may result in limitations in craniocaudal mobility. In addition, the lateral approach may be prevented by the pelvis and organs of the thorax and abdomen. Furthermore, structures exerting posterior compression on the spinal canal cannot be reached with the transforaminal access, so its use is limited for stenoses within the spinal canal. Foraminal stenoses in the sense of superior articular process (SAP) impingement with cranial compression of the exiting spinal nerves can be decompressed. In this case, an extraforaminal approach can also be selected that allows entry into the foramen under view.

Because of the limitations of the transforaminal approach, the full-endoscopic interlaminar approach was developed, which makes it possible to operate on pathologic conditions located within the spinal canal that are beyond the range of indications for the transforaminal approach.[10,11] Today, lateral and central spinal canal stenoses and intraspinal extradural cysts can be decompressed in a full-endoscopic interlaminar technique, also bilaterally in an over-the-top technique with a unilateral approach[12–14] (**Fig. 1**).

INDICATIONS/CONTRAINDICATIONS

The indication for surgery must be made according to today's standard based on radicular symptoms, neurogenic claudication, and existing neurologic deficits.[15,16] Isolated back pain cannot usually be improved by decompressive operations. Existing secondary pathologic conditions, such as instabilities, may have to be treated at the same time using other procedures. It must be planned preoperatively whether, depending on the anatomy and pathologic condition, the transforaminal/extraforaminal or interlaminar access for decompression can be used. The following indications are currently unequivocal.

Indications

- Lumbar degenerative lateral and central spinal canal stenosis
- Intraspinal and intraforaminal/extraforaminal extradural cysts

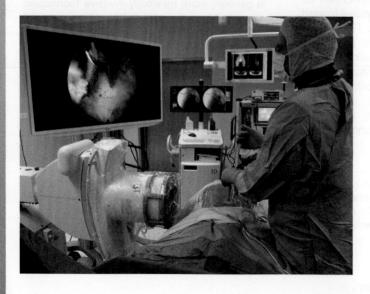

Fig. 1. Setup with a full-endoscopic interlaminar approach.

- Corresponding radicular symptoms and/or corresponding neurogenic claudication with or without neurologic deficits
- Conservative treatment, unsuccessful or not, indicated based on the symptoms

Contraindications

- Back pain as a main symptom
- Instability/deformities with an indication for a stabilizing procedure

SURGICAL TECHNIQUE/PROCEDURE
Preoperative planning

The preoperative preparation is the same as the preparation for conventional, microsurgical operations. The intraoperative procedure must be planned preoperatively based on imaging findings. The goal is to perform the resection of spinal canal structures as sparingly as possible depending on the pathologic condition. Conventional 2-plane radiographs of the lumbar spine and MRI with sagittal and transverse reconstruction are obligatory. In applying the lateral transforaminal approach, the access pathway may not be shifted by abdominal structures. Therefore, in the lateral transforaminal approach, an abdominal computed tomographic (CT) scan or wide-view lumbar CT or MRI may be necessary to verify that intraabdominal structures are not in the path of the planned surgical trajectory. No additional examinations specifically for full-endoscopic operations are necessary.

Preparation and patient positioning

The operations are performed with the patient in prone position on a radiograph-permeable table, under orthograde 2-plane fluoroscopic control. The patient lies on a hip and thorax roll to relieve the abdominal and thoracic organs to alleviate epidural bleeding. The operating table can be adjusted for lordosis or kyphosis intraoperatively at the lumbar level, depending on the anatomy and pathologic condition. In every procedure, a single-shot antibiosis is applied for infection prophylaxis.

SURGICAL APPROACH AND PROCEDURE
Lateral Transforaminal/Extraforaminal Approach

- The position of the skin incision is determined under lateral and posterior-anterior (p.a). radiological control. The operative goal is to reach the spinal canal as close to the coronal plane as possible without injuring abdominal organs.

Transforaminal approach

- A spinal needle is inserted orthograde to the disc space into the target region, typically the dorsal aspect of the disc space at the junction of the posterior longitudinal ligament and annulus. A guide wire is introduced,and the needle is removed. The dilator is inserted, and the working sheath is advanced over the dilator. From this point, decompression is performed under visualization and continuous irrigation.
- The endoscope is withdrawn, and the foramen is dissected, that is, the ascending facet joint, the disc, and, if applicable, the exiting spinal nerve.

Extraforaminal approach

- If the position of the exiting nerve is not clear, an extraforaminal approach can be performed. For this, the spinal needle is placed on the caudal pedicle (**Fig. 2**).
- Then, the foramen is dissected, and the needle may be passed through the foramen under visualization.

Decompression of lateral recess stenosis

- Bone resection at the ascending facet until the medial edge of the facet can be reached over the entire extension of the stenosis.
- The medial edge of the ascending facet joint is resected along with any attached segments of the ligamentum flavum (**Fig. 3**).
- Stenotic segments of the annulus may also be resected.

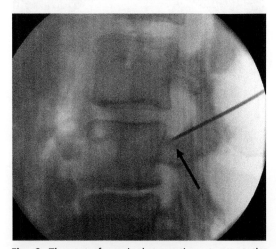

Fig. 2. The extraforaminal operation starts at the caudal pedicle. (*arrow*, final position of spinal needle).

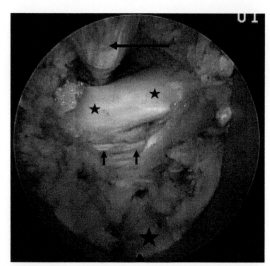

Fig. 3. View into the spinal canal after transforaminal decompression. (*large arrow*, bipolar electrode; *small stars*, spinal nerve; *small arrows*, posterior longitudinal ligament; *large star*, disc space).

Decompression of a foraminal stenosis (superior articular process impingement)

- The cranial tip of the ascending facet joint is visualized (**Fig. 4**).
- Preserving the exiting spinal nerve, the tip of the facet joint is resected with any attached segments of the ligamentum flavum until the exiting spinal nerve is no longer compressed.

Interlaminar Approach

- The position of the skin incision for a posterior approach is determined under posterior-anterior (p.a). fluoroscopic guidance as medial as possible over the interlaminar window.
- The dilator is inserted bluntly, and the working sheath is advanced over the dilator under fluoroscopic guidance. From this point, decompression is performed under visualization and continuous irrigation.
- The ligamentum flavum and adjacent bony structures of the interlaminar window are dissected, and the vertebral joint is opened to visualize the caudal tip of the descending facet joint.

Decompression of lateral recess stenosis

- Ipsilateral resection of the descending facet, the cranial, and the caudal lamina until the over the entire length of compression. Resection is generally continued cranially until the tip of the ascending facet joint is reached and caudally to the middle of the pedicle (**Figs. 5** and **6**).
- The ligamentum flavum and any other bony structures or the annulus are resected until the ipsilateral side is decompressed (**Fig. 7**).

Decompression of a central stenosis

- For mobility of the contralateral side, the lamina and anterior region of the spinous processes are resected until sufficient space has been made to reach the contralateral

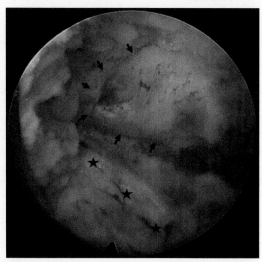

Fig. 4. The cranial tip of the ascending facet (*arrows*) and the exiting spinal nerve (*stars*) in SAP impingement.

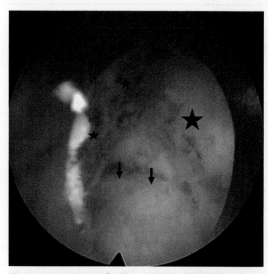

Fig. 5. Resection of the medial descending facet (*small stars*) until the corresponding joint surface can be seen and the cranial tip of the ascending facet (*arrows*) is reached (*large star*, flavum ligament).

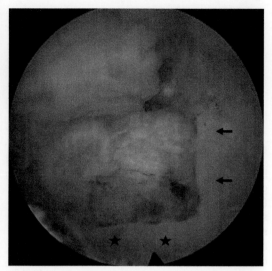

Fig. 6. Bone resection at the medial edge of the ascending facet (*stars*) and the caudal lamina (*arrows*) up to the middle of the caudal pedicle.

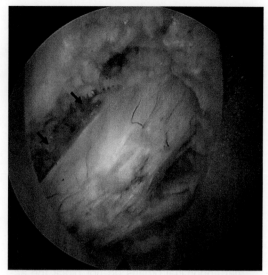

Fig. 8. Bilateral over-the-top decompression with an ipsilateral approach for central stenosis. (*arrows*, contralateral decompression).

side in the over-the-top technique posterior to the cauda equina without pressing the endoscope against the neural structures.

- The working cannula is then angled toward the contralateral side to perform the "over-the-top" resection of the contralateral ligamentum flavum and any compressing bony structures (**Fig. 8**).
- The contralateral neural structures should not be shifted in the medial direction for decompression in the anterior region because of the high risk of compression of the cauda equina.

COMPLICATIONS AND MANAGEMENT

Possible complications during microsurgical procedures are known, and there is a wide body of literature on this subject. In principle, all the complications known from conventional operating procedures may occur.

- Intraoperative complications: for example, surgery on the wrong segment, epidural bleeding, insufficient decompression, injuries to the dura, injuries to neural structures, injuries to vessels, injuries to organs
- Direct postoperative complications: for example, persistent or progressive radicular symptoms, cauda equina syndrome, urinary retention, consequences of injury to vessels or organs
- Delayed postoperative complications: soft tissue infection, spondylodiscitis, cerebrospinal fluid fistula, delayed consequences of injury to vessels or organs, further radicular symptoms, surgically induced symptoms (failed back surgery syndrome)

With respect to the full-endoscopic technique, the following points in particular must be taken into consideration:

- In the interlaminar approach, a long-lasting and uninterrupted excessive retraction of the neural structures with the working sheath in medial direction must be avoided or be only intermittent in order to avoid the risk of neurologic damage.

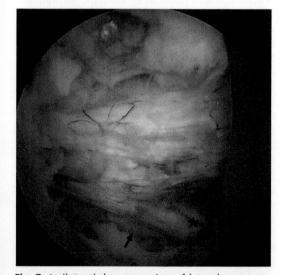

Fig. 7. Ipsilateral decompression of lateral recess stenosis (*star*, spinal nerve; *arrows*, lateral recess).

- If the dura is injured, direct suturing in the full-endoscopic technique is possible in some cases. Otherwise, the injury can be covered with dura substitute, fibrin glue, or an additional fat flap. An intraoperative switch to an open procedure should be considered only for very large dura defects.
- In the transforaminal approach, the risk of injury to the exiting nerves cannot be completely eliminated. The highest risk occurs while performing the approach itself. If the risk is to be avoided, it is necessary to remain strictly within the caudal aspect of the foramen. Alternatively, if the foramen is narrowed, an extraforaminal approach should be performed if necessary.
- When the lateral transforaminal/extraforaminal access is used, it is important to ensure that abdominal organs do not block the access path. It is particularly important to take this into account at the levels cranial to L4-5.
- Theoretically, if operating times are extended and blockage for outflow of irrigation fluid is overlooked, the consequences of increased pressure within the spinal canal and the attached and neighboring structures cannot be completely ruled out. Operations should therefore be performed leaving the system open so that the irrigation fluid can flow out.
- Especially during the learning curve, experience has shown that there is an increased risk of complications occurring, as with any new technique. Prior observation of and assistance in procedures and workshops involving practice on cadavers might well be instructive.

POSTOPERATIVE CARE

- The length of the hospital stay depends on the operative measures. Pure discectomies or simple decompressions are treated in brief hospitalization or, if patient care at home is adequate, on an outpatient basis.
- Mobilization is immediate, as soon as anesthesia allows.
- No operation-related pain medication is required.
- Except for patients with neurologic deficits, no rehabilitative measures are necessary. Isometric and coordinative exercises can be performed without supervision once they are learned. A passive lumbar brace during the day is prescribed for about 6 weeks. The load level can be increased depending on the pathologic condition and subjective well-being.
- Return to work and sports is possible under the same conditions after wound healing. Limitations are imposed only in that there should be no increase in pain under the activity. After more extensive operations, the postsurgical treatment regimen is usually more restrictive and depends on the individual intervention performed.

OUTCOMES

In general, the available literature reports mainly good clinical outcomes and low complication rates for endoscopic lumbar decompression, although study results for disc herniation and spinal canal stenosis must also be taken into consideration.[10,17–20] On the 1 hand, studies show that no differences were found in the results between endoscopic and microsurgical procedures.[18,21,22] In a review, the overall evidence for an advantage of the more minimally invasive procedure compared with open procedures is criticized.[23] On the other hand, advantages have been reported for endoscopy, for example, with respect to the clinical outcome, complications, shorter operation times, shorter hospital stay, or faster rehabilitation.[24–27] A comparison of the results is sometimes limited because various operative approaches are used with different indications that are still not standardized today. Despite the perceptible increase in relevant studies, there is still a need for high-quality comparison studies, especially on the direct comparison with microsurgical techniques.[23]

With respect to possible operation-induced negative consequences and potential complications, the same discussions about microsurgical procedures also apply to endoscopic techniques. The general rate of complications is reported with a range of 2.9% to 13.75%, for example.[28–30] Here, also, a comparison is sometimes difficult because complications and study designs are not always uniform. Dura injuries occur in literature with rates ranging from 0% to around 5%,[25,29,31–33] and nerve injuries occur at rates from 0% to around 2.5%.[10,21,29,34] In a transforaminal approach, there may be a higher risk for damage to the exiting nerve during access, which is why some investigators prefer to perform the procedure under local anesthesia.[35,36] Overall, according to a metaanalysis, there is a lower rate of complications than with a microsurgical procedure.[29] No infections or operation-induced instabilities were reported in the literature.[25] In a metaanalysis, other complications (eg, wrong level, general medical complications, hematoma, wound problems) were reported to be 1.1%, lower than in a microsurgical procedure.[29]

One particular difficulty for newer, more technical procedures is the learning curve, because higher complication rates cannot be ruled out during this time. In general, the learning curve for full-endoscopic disc operations has been described as relatively steep, so that stable outcomes can be achieved after an acceptable number of cases.[30,37–39] Studies report that the learning curve is completed after 40 cases for the interlaminar approach, 17 cases for the transforaminal approach, or 10 to 20 cases without exact differentiation of the approach.[40–42] In general, the learning curve appears to be difficult, but not unusually so and is within the range of the learning curve for laparoscopic procedures.[43,44]

SUMMARY

- The full-endoscopic lumbar technique for operating spinal canal stenoses is used today as a largely standard procedure and allows sufficient decompression.
- For the transforaminal/extraforaminal approach, there are clear inclusion and exclusion criteria and thus also limitations, so the full-endoscopic interlaminar approach is usually used for the decompression of lateral and central spinal canal stenoses.
- Full-endoscopic techniques can have advantages and can be used as an alternative to a microsurgical procedure.

REFERENCES

1. Mayer HM, List J, Korge A, et al. [Microsurgery of acquired degenerative lumbar spinal stenosis. Bilateral over-the-top decompression through unilateral approach]. Orthopade 2003;32(10):889–95.
2. Ragab AA, Fye MA, Bohlman HH. Surgery of the lumbar spine for spinal stenosis in 118 patients 70 years of age or older. Spine (Phila Pa 1976) 2003; 28(4):348–53.
3. Silverplats K, Lind B, Zoega B, et al. Health-related quality of life in patients with surgically treated lumbar disc herniation: 2- and 7-year follow-up of 117 patients. Acta Orthop 2011;82(2):198–203.
4. Daniell JR, Osti OL. Failed back surgery syndrome: a review article. Asian Spine J 2018;12(2):372–9.
5. Goald HJ. Microlumbar discectomy: followup of 147 patients. Spine (Phila Pa 1976) 1978;3(2):183–5.
6. Schick U, Dohnert J, Richter A, et al. Microendoscopic lumbar discectomy versus open surgery: an intraoperative EMG study. Eur Spine J 2002; 11(1):20–6.
7. Ruetten S, Komp M, Godolias G. An extreme lateral access for the surgery of lumbar disc herniations inside the spinal canal using the full-endoscopic uniportal transforaminal approach–technique and prospective results of 463 patients. Spine (Phila Pa 1976) 2005;30(22):2570–8.
8. Kambin P, Casey K, O'Brien E, et al. Transforaminal arthroscopic decompression of lateral recess stenosis. J Neurosurg 1996;84(3):462–7.
9. Mayer HM, Brock M. Percutaneous endoscopic discectomy: surgical technique and preliminary results compared to microsurgical discectomy. J Neurosurg 1993;78(2):216–25.
10. Ruetten S, Komp M, Merk H, et al. Full-endoscopic interlaminar and transforaminal lumbar discectomy versus conventional microsurgical technique: a prospective, randomized, controlled study. Spine (Phila Pa 1976) 2008;33(9):931–9.
11. Ruetten S, Komp M, Godolias G. A new full-endoscopic technique for the interlaminar operation of lumbar disc herniations using 6-mm endoscopes: prospective 2-year results of 331 patients. Minim Invasive Neurosurg 2006;49(2):80–7.
12. Komp M, Hahn P, Oezdemir S, et al. Bilateral spinal decompression of lumbar central stenosis with the full-endoscopic interlaminar versus microsurgical laminotomy technique: a prospective, randomized, controlled study. Pain Physician 2015; 18(1):61–70.
13. Komp M, Hahn P, Ozdemir S, et al. Operation of lumbar zygoapophyseal joint cysts using a full-endoscopic interlaminar and transforaminal approach: prospective 2-year results of 74 patients. Surg Innov 2014;21(6):605–14.
14. Ruetten S, Komp M, Merk H, et al. Surgical treatment for lumbar lateral recess stenosis with the full-endoscopic interlaminar approach versus conventional microsurgical technique: a prospective, randomized, controlled study. J Neurosurg Spine 2009;10(5):476–85.
15. Andersson GB, Brown MD, Dvorak J, et al. Consensus summary of the diagnosis and treatment of lumbar disc herniation. Spine (Phila Pa 1976) 1996;21(24 Suppl):75S–8S.
16. McCulloch JA. Focus issue on lumbar disc herniation: macro- and microdiscectomy. Spine (Phila Pa 1976) 1996;21(24 Suppl):45S–56S.
17. Chen HC, Lee CH, Wei L, et al. Comparison of percutaneous endoscopic lumbar discectomy and open lumbar surgery for adjacent segment degeneration and recurrent disc herniation. Neurol Res Int 2015;2015:791943.
18. Chen Z, Zhang L, Dong J, et al. Percutaneous transforaminal endoscopic discectomy compared with microendoscopic discectomy for lumbar disc herniation: 1-year results of an ongoing randomized controlled trial. J Neurosurg Spine 2018;28(3): 300–10.
19. Nakamura JI, Yoshihara K. Initial clinical outcomes of percutaneous full-endoscopic lumbar discectomy

using an interlaminar approach at the L4-L5. Pain Physician 2017;20(4):E507–12.

20. Phan K, Xu J, Schultz K, et al. Full-endoscopic versus micro-endoscopic and open discectomy: a systematic review and meta-analysis of outcomes and complications. Clin Neurol Neurosurg 2017; 154:1–12.

21. Casimiro M. Short-term outcome comparison between full-endoscopic interlaminar approach and open minimally invasive microsurgical technique for treatment of lumbar disc herniation. World Neurosurg 2017;108:894–900.e1.

22. Kamper SJ, Ostelo RW, Rubinstein SM, et al. Minimally invasive surgery for lumbar disc herniation: a systematic review and meta-analysis. Eur Spine J 2014;23(5):1021–43.

23. Evaniew N, Khan M, Drew B, et al. Minimally invasive versus open surgery for cervical and lumbar discectomy: a systematic review and meta-analysis. CMAJ Open 2014;2(4):E295–305.

24. Feng F, Xu Q, Yan F, et al. Comparison of 7 surgical interventions for lumbar disc herniation: a network meta-analysis. Pain Physician 2017;20(6):E863–71.

25. Liu X, Yuan S, Tian Y, et al. Comparison of percutaneous endoscopic transforaminal discectomy, microendoscopic discectomy, and microdiscectomy for symptomatic lumbar disc herniation: minimum 2-year follow-up results. J Neurosurg Spine 2018; 28(3):317–25.

26. Ruetten S, Komp M, Merk H, et al. Full-endoscopic cervical posterior foraminotomy for the operation of lateral disc herniations using 5.9-mm endoscopes: a prospective, randomized, controlled study. Spine (Phila Pa 1976) 2008;33(9):940–8.

27. Tu Z, Li YW, Wang B, et al. Clinical outcome of full-endoscopic interlaminar discectomy for single-level lumbar disc herniation: a minimum of 5-year follow-up. Pain Physician 2017;20(3):E425–30.

28. Li X, Chang H, Meng X. Tubular microscopes discectomy versus conventional microdiscectomy for treating lumbar disk herniation: systematic review and meta-analysis. Medicine (Baltimore) 2018; 97(5):e9807.

29. Shriver MF, Xie JJ, Tye EY, et al. Lumbar microdiscectomy complication rates: a systematic review and meta-analysis. Neurosurg Focus 2015;39(4):E6.

30. Xie TH, Zeng JC, Li ZH, et al. Complications of lumbar disc herniation following full-endoscopic interlaminar lumbar discectomy: a large, single-center, retrospective study. Pain Physician 2017;20(3): E379–87.

31. Nie H, Zeng J, Song Y, et al. Percutaneous endoscopic lumbar discectomy for L5-S1 disc herniation via an interlaminar approach versus a transforaminal approach: a prospective randomized controlled study with 2-year follow up. Spine (Phila Pa 1976) 2016;41(Suppl 19):B30–7.

32. Ruetten S, Komp M, Merk H, et al. Use of newly developed instruments and endoscopes: full-endoscopic resection of lumbar disc herniations via the interlaminar and lateral transforaminal approach. J Neurosurg Spine 2007;6(6):521–30.

33. Song H, Hu W, Liu Z, et al. Percutaneous endoscopic interlaminar discectomy of L5-S1 disc herniation: a comparison between intermittent endoscopy technique and full endoscopy technique. J Orthop Surg Res 2017;12(1):162.

34. Yorukoglu AG, Goker B, Tahta A, et al. Fully endoscopic interlaminar and transforaminal lumbar discectomy: analysis of 47 complications encountered in a series of 835 patients. Neurocirugia (Astur) 2017;28(5):235–41.

35. Sairyo K, Chikawa T, Nagamachi A. State-of-the-art transforaminal percutaneous endoscopic lumbar surgery under local anesthesia: discectomy, foraminoplasty, and ventral facetectomy. J Orthop Sci 2018;23(2):229–36.

36. Shin SH, Bae JS, Lee SH, et al. Transforaminal endoscopic decompression for lumbar spinal stenosis: a novel surgical technique and clinical outcomes. World Neurosurg 2018;114:e873–82.

37. Hsu HT, Chang SJ, Yang SS, et al. Learning curve of full-endoscopic lumbar discectomy. Eur Spine J 2013;22(4):727–33.

38. Passacantilli E, Lenzi J, Caporlingua F, et al. Endoscopic interlaminar approach for intracanal L5-S1 disc herniation: classification of disc prolapse in relation to learning curve and surgical outcome. Asian J Endosc Surg 2015;8(4):445–53.

39. Xu H, Liu X, Liu G, et al. Learning curve of full-endoscopic technique through interlaminar approach for L5/S1 disk herniations. Cell Biochem Biophys 2014;70(2):1069–74.

40. Joswig H, Richter H, Haile SR, et al. Introducing interlaminar full-endoscopic lumbar diskectomy: a critical analysis of complications, recurrence rates, and outcome in view of two spinal surgeons' learning curves. J Neurol Surg A Cent Eur Neurosurg 2016;77(5):406–15.

41. Lee DY, Lee SH. Learning curve for percutaneous endoscopic lumbar discectomy. Neurol Med Chir (Tokyo) 2008;48(9):383–8 [discussion: 388–9].

42. Wang B, Lu G, Patel AA, et al. An evaluation of the learning curve for a complex surgical technique: the full endoscopic interlaminar approach for lumbar disc herniations. Spine J 2011;11(2):122–30.

43. Kim Y, Lee W. The learning curve of single-port laparoscopic appendectomy performed by emergent operation. World J Emerg Surg 2016;11:39.

44. Tay CW, Shen L, Hartman M, et al. SILC for SILC: single institution learning curve for single-incision laparoscopic cholecystectomy. Minim Invasive Surg 2013;2013:381628.

Lateral Lumbar Interbody Fusion

Houtan A. Taba, MD, Seth K. Williams, MD*

KEYWORDS

- OLIF • XLIF • DLIF • Lateral • Lumbar • Spine • MIS

KEY POINTS

- Lateral lumbar interbody fusion has powerful indirect decompression capacity due to large footprint of cage-spanning apophyses.
- Deformity correction with lateral lumbar interbody fusion has shown significant coronal correction and when used in conjunction with other techniques can significantly improve sagittal deformity as well.
- New applications in treatment of infection, trauma, and tumor show promise for purposes of debridement, decompression, and stabilization through an anteriorly based procedure from the lateral approach.
- Lateral instrumentation and stand-alone procedures are sufficient for some pathology and capable of reducing surgical time and complications.

INTRODUCTION

The retroperitoneal lateral lumbar interbody fusion (LLIF) technique is increasingly used for the treatment of a variety of lumbar spinal conditions. First described by McAfee and colleagues[1] in 1998 and later elaborated on by Ozgur and colleagues[2] in 2006, the direct lateral transpsoas technique introduced a new approach to the anterior column that facilitated the placement of relatively large footprint interbody cages through a minimally invasive muscle-sparing approach. Anterior-to-psoas (ATP), also called prepsoas, lateral approaches also were developed during this period, first described by Mayer in 1997.[3] The transpsoas and ATP approaches represent the 2 surgical corridors for performing the retroperitoneal lateral lumbar fusion, with some variation in approach nuances and related risks and morbidity.

Here we aim to review the LLIF technique in the treatment of various lumbar spinal pathologies, with a discussion of outcomes, approach-related complications associated specific to the lateral technique, and areas of new research.

INDICATIONS FOR LATERAL LUMBAR INTERBODY FUSION

One of the most popular indications for LLIF is indirect decompression of the neural elements by restoring a collapsed disk height or correcting spondylolisthesis or scoliosis by placement of the interbody cage. Placement of an interbody cage across the apophyses in the lumbar disk space has been shown in several studies to significantly increase foraminal cross-sectional area, central canal cross-sectional area, and disk height.[4–7] This has particular advantages in revision surgery, when an open decompression has a relatively high durotomy rate, whereas a durotomy during a lateral fusion operation is highly unusual.[8]

Disclosure Statement: S.K. Williams: Consultant: DePuy Synthes Spine, Stryker Spine. Stock ownership: Titan Spine.
Department of Orthopedics and Rehabilitation, University of Wisconsin – Madison, Madison, WI, USA
* Corresponding author. 4602 East Park Boulevard, Madison, WI 53718.
E-mail address: swilliams@ortho.wisc.edu

Neurosurg Clin N Am 31 (2020) 33–42
https://doi.org/10.1016/j.nec.2019.08.004
1042-3680/20/© 2019 Elsevier Inc. All rights reserved.

neurosurgery.theclinics.com

The lateral approach has utility beyond degenerative or deformity circumstances. As experience with the LLIF techniques has increased, publications have shown effective use of the lateral approach in the treatment of infectious, neoplastic, and traumatic thoracolumbar conditions.

TECHNIQUE AND PERTINENT ANATOMY

The lateral retroperitoneal approach to the lumbar spine can be subdivided into 2 techniques with regard to management of the psoas. Proprietary names for the transpsoas technique include the "direct lateral interbody fusion" (DLIF), and the "extreme lateral interbody fusion" (XLIF), and an ATP technique may be called an "oblique lateral interbody fusion" (OLIF). These techniques usually allow for access of the lumbar spine from the L1/2 to the L4/5 disk space. The patient is placed in a lateral decubitus position typically with the left side up and prepped and draped in a sterile fashion. Fluoroscopy or image guidance is used to plan the skin incision. The retroperitoneal space is then accessed by dividing the fascia and muscle layers of the external oblique, internal oblique and transverse abdominal muscles. Blunt dissection is then performed to sweep the peritoneum anteriorly to identify the psoas muscle. The disc space is identified and can be accessed anterior to the psoas or trans-psoas depending on surgeon preference.

LUMBAR DEFORMITY

Many studies demonstrate significant coronal plane deformity correction and improvement in outcome measures in the short and long term with the utilization of the LLIF technique for adult spinal deformity.[9,10] An additional advantage of LLIF for the treatment of adult spinal deformity is the potential to achieve similar global deformity correction over fewer spinal segments secondary to the anterior column support from the large interbody placed through the lateral retroperitoneal corridor (**Fig. 1**).[11] For a lumbar degenerative curve, it is often possible to perform a 2-level or 3-level lateral interbody fusion with posterior percutaneous instrumentation rather than an open posterior T10-ilum fusion. Traditional deformity procedures are large operations with significant blood loss, approach-related muscle trauma, long hospital stays, and complication rates of 30% or greater.[12] In addition to the powerful deformity correction associated with the utilization of the minimally invasive LLIF technique, it avoids the risks of the large traditional posteriorly based deformity procedures.[11] Uribe and colleagues[13] compared complications of minimally invasive LLIF with hybrid and open procedures for adult spinal deformity and reported substantially less blood loss and a lower complication rate with similar improvements in outcomes.

A potential disadvantage in the treatment of adult spinal deformity through LLIF techniques alone is the limited ability to achieve significant sagittal plane correction.[10] Sagittal plane correction is a primary objective in adult spinal deformity surgery. However, utilization of LLIF in combination with open posterior techniques has been shown to improve coronal and sagittal plane correction comparable to traditional posterior techniques alone, while incurring a lower complication rate.[14–16]

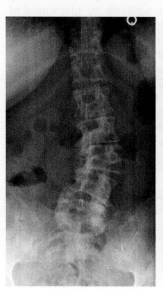 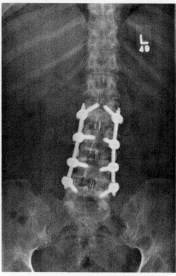

Fig. 1. An additional advantage of LLIF for the treatment of adult spinal deformity is the potential to achieve similar global deformity correction over fewer spinal segments secondary to the anterior column support from the interbody cage placed through the lateral retroperitoneal corridor. Pre-operative AP radiograph showing lumbar degenerative scoliosis (*Left*). Post-operative AP radiograph after a 3-level lateral interbody fusion showing complete coronal plane deformity correction (*Right*).

Recently, the anterior column realignment (ACR) procedure has been described as a laterally based interbody fusion technique with greater capacity for sagittal deformity correction. In the ACR procedure, the anterior longitudinal ligament (ALL) is sharply released. The ALL is typically preserved in LLIF, as it provides a restraint to anterior migration of the cage as well as resistance for tensioning of the interbody cage. In the management of deformity with significant sagittal plane involvement, release of the ALL has been performed to enhance sagittal correction. ALL release has shown sagittal plane correction even greater than that of pedicle subtraction osteotomy with substantially less surgical time and blood loss.[17,18] Release of the ALL through the lateral approach requires significant preoperative study of the vascular anatomy as major vessel injury is a risk of ACR, but this can be reduced with planning and experience (**Fig. 2**).

LUMBAR DEGENERATIVE CONDITIONS

Recent literature shows treatment of a variety of degenerative conditions with LLIF can result in improvement in back pain and lower extremity pain. This includes the treatment of degenerative disk disease with foraminal and central stenosis, degenerative spondylolisthesis with or without stenosis and adjacent segment degeneration.[19–24] The treatment of spondylolisthesis is a common indication for LLIF. Studies have shown improvement in clinical outcomes and partial to complete reduction in both Meyerding grade I

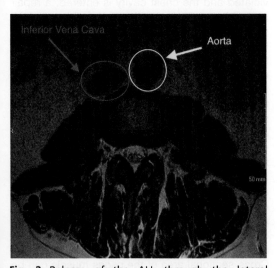

Fig. 2. Release of the ALL through the lateral approach requires diligent preoperative study of the vascular anatomy as major vessel injury is a risk of ACR, but this can be reduced with planning and experience.

and grade II spondylolisthesis.[20,21,25] Sato and colleagues[20] also demonstrated indirect decompression in spondylolisthesis, reporting improvements in axial and sagittal canal diameter, cross-sectional area of the spinal canal, and increased disk height and foraminal area. Although short-term results for the treatment of spondylolisthesis with LLIF show improvement in radiographic parameters and clinical outcomes, longer-term studies are necessary to show maintained improvement.

LUMBAR ADJACENT SEGMENT DISEASE

Adjacent segment disease (ASD) is the development of symptomatic degeneration of the spine adjacent to a previously fused segment. This can include disk degeneration, listhesis, instability, hypertrophic facet joint arthrosis, focal scoliosis, herniated nucleus pulposus, and stenosis.[26] Lateral surgery for the treatment of ASD is appealing, because when performed on a standalone basis, with or without lateral plating, the morbidity of a revision posterior approach can be avoided. In addition, ASD has been hypothesized to be exacerbated by disruption of the posterior ligamentous structures and tension band.[27] Similarly, laminectomy alone adjacent to a fusion construct can further destabilize the spine leading to a high risk for recurrent ASD.[28] A retrospective series of patients with ASD treated with LLIF reported improvement in clinical and radiographic outcomes in patients treated with both standalone LLIF and circumferential fusion.[24] Standalone LLIF has been hypothesized to be sufficient for the treatment of ASD where dynamic instability is not present.[29] A recent study of standalone LLIF showed clinical and radiographic improvement over 18 months of postoperative follow-up with only a 12% reoperation rate for addition of posterior instrumentation.[30]

LATERAL APPROACH FOR INFECTION, TRAUMA, AND NEOPLASTIC DISEASE

Patients presenting with lumbar trauma, diskitis/osteomyelitis, or metastatic disease share some common characteristics. They typically present acutely and are often not medically optimized for surgery, making minimally invasive surgical approaches particularly appealing in an effort to minimize the risk of complications. As the minimally invasive lateral technique has increased in adoption, there are reports of management of infection, trauma, and neoplastic disease with the lateral approach. Many of these conditions historically have required extensive posterior approaches and avoiding approach-related morbidity in these populations is of great value.

There is a growing body of literature showing promise in treatment of lumbar diskitis/osteomyelitis through a lateral approach. Many cases of diskitis/osteomyelitis can be treated with systemic antibiotics alone, but some infections are recalcitrant or inappropriate to manage medically. Often patients with diskitis/osteomyelitis have comorbid conditions leading to an increased risk for complications from an open posterior technique. Two case series and a case report of the lateral approach for debridement and stabilization are available in the literature. These studies demonstrated effective eradication of infection and no failures of debridement during the follow-up periods.[31-33]

Less has been published regarding the treatment of primary and metastatic neoplastic disease of the spine through a lateral approach. However, there are reports of tumor resection and stabilization through the lateral technique.[34-36] Utilization of a lateral approach for treatment avoids the more extensive midline posterior incision, which may reduce the risk of wound complications and allow for a shorter delay to initiation of chemotherapy and radiation if appropriate.

For treatment of thoracolumbar trauma, the lateral approach can be used to perform anterior decompression and placement of an interbody cage. This provides direct neural element decompression and anterior stabilization that allows for sagittal alignment correction. Supplemental lateral plating or posterior percutaneous pedicle screw placement creates a biomechanically stronger construct compared with posterior pedicle screw placement alone.[37] Recent case series have demonstrated effective treatment of thoracolumbar trauma through the lateral approach with or without posterior instrumentation.[36-38]

ADVANCED CONSIDERATIONS

Anterior and posterior techniques for interbody fusion of the lumbar spine sacrifice stabilizing ligamentous and bony structures, often necessitating supplemental fixation. The lateral interbody fusion technique preserves the ALL, posterior longitudinal ligament, and the posterior elements. As a result of the preserved stabilizers, surgeons have expanded indications for stand-alone LLIF, meaning no supplemental fixation either lateral or posterior. The reported indications for consideration of stand-alone LLIF include degenerative disk disease, low-grade stable degenerative spondylolisthesis, and adjacent segment degeneration. Malham and colleagues[39] proposed an algorithm with which candidates for stand-alone XLIF procedures could be identified, and patients were prospectively assigned to a stand-alone construct or supplemental fixation. They found no subsidence with larger 22-mm depth cages but did encounter subsidence with 18-mm depth cages.[39] Other studies have shown similar findings.[40] Biomechanical studies of stand-alone LLIF show stability that compares favorably with other interbody fusions with adjunctive posterior fixation.[41,42] Ultimately, the decision to proceed with stand-alone LLIF should be made on a case-by-case basis, and does carry some risk of cage subsidence compared with lateral constructs with adjunctive fixation. Healthy, thin, nonsmoking patients with good bone quality and 1 or 2-level pathology may be considered for stand-alone LLIF if a large footprint interbody is placed and the underlying pathology does not involve significant instability.[39,43]

As mentioned previously, the LLIF procedure allows access from the L1/2 level to the L4/5 level. Both extremes pose challenges during the approach. At the L1/2 level, if the conus or spinal cord are present, an indirect decompression may pose an increased risk for neurologic injury, and consideration for an open posterior procedure in severe stenosis should be considered.[44] Because of the cephalad location, with L1/2 and sometimes L2/3, a rib may be present in the desired approach trajectory necessitating a partial rib resection. Care should be taken to avoid injury to the subcostal nerve along the inferior border of the rib. Deeper in the approach, the diaphragm is present, if violated and the chest cavity is entered, a repair should be performed with the possible need for placement of a chest tube. Caudally at the L4/5 level there are 3 main anatomic considerations that may make access to the disk space more difficult. These are the iliac crest relationship to the L4/5 disk space, the vascular anatomy, and the larger diameter of the psoas. If the L4/5 disk space is at the level of or cephalad to the iliac crest, then the iliac crest should not present a substantial impediment to accessing the disk space from a lateral trajectory. If the iliac crest is cephalad to the L4/5 disk space, access becomes more difficult, although may be facilitated by curved, angled, and offset instruments. The anteroposterior radiograph should be scrutinized to determine if obliquity is present that may lead to a more favorable access from a particular side. Cross-sectional area of the psoas muscle can be assessed on MRI or computed tomography (CT) scan. At the L4/5 level in some patients, the psoas can be quite large (**Fig. 3**). This may represent a relative contraindication to the lateral approach,

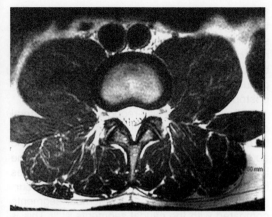

Fig. 3. Cross-sectional area of the psoas muscle can be assessed on MRI or CT scan. At the L4/5 level in some patients, the psoas can be quite large.

as there is an increased risk of muscle injury and possibly lumbar plexus injury. At the L4/5 level, a more anteriorly positioned psoas muscle has been hypothesized to lead to increased risk of neurologic injury, whereas other studies suggest a larger psoas cross-sectional area may have a protective effect.[45,46] The vascular anatomy also should be scrutinized at the L4/5 level, especially when considering a right-sided approach because the iliac vein may be overlying the disk space. The iliolumbar vein is potentially at risk as well at L4/5.

Intraoperative neuromonitoring (IONM) through dynamic evoked electromyography is recommended for safe performance of a transpsoas LLIF.[47] The risk for nerve injury increases caudally in the lumbar spine as the lumbar plexus is more anteriorly located in the psoas. Although safe zones have been described, IONM continues to be recommended to reduce the risk of lumbar plexus injury. Recent literature has questioned the necessity of IONM when LLIF is to be accomplished at single levels cephalad to L4/5 and if the surgeon emphasizes a more atraumatic technique with effort at direct visualization of the plexus about the psoas.[48] An experienced lateral surgeon may consider forgoing IONM in an effort to minimize surgical time, as a component of neurologic findings are thought to be related to ischemic injury from prolonged retractor deployment time.

Supplemental posterior fixation enhances stability in LLIF procedures. Traditionally, percutaneous pedicle screw placement and other posterior instrumentation is performed with the patient in the prone position. This requires repositioning the patient during surgery, which adds time and the possibility of complications from removal of tubes or lines during the repositioning. Investigators have reported on the feasibility of posterior instrumentation in the lateral position for placement of pedicle screws or transfacet screws (**Fig. 4**).[49–52] These studies showed no compromise in lordosis with posterior fixation with the

A 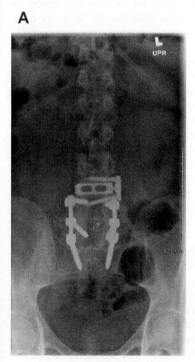   **B**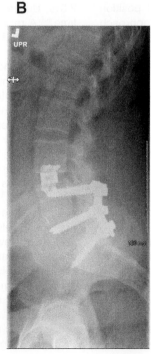

Fig. 4. Post-operative AP (*A*) and lateral (*B*) radiographs showing treatment of adjacent segment disease with L3/4 LLIF and supplemental lateral plating, above a previous L4-S1 posterior instrumented fusion construct.

patient in the lateral decubitus position and no increase in complication rates. With experience, surgeons can consider performing posterior instrumentation in the lateral decubitus position. In the authors' experience, this is best considered in patients who are thin, have good bone quality, and favorable pedicle diameter and trajectory.

CT-based navigation techniques are known to reduce radiation exposure to the surgical team and allow for reliable implant positioning. Minimally invasive techniques are typically fluoroscopy-dependent due to the lack of direct visualization of patient anatomy. Surgeons have described techniques using CT-based navigation to perform LLIF procedures.[53–56] Benefits in the LLIF for navigation include allowing for precise incision localization, reducing incision length, and minimizing soft-tissue disturbance. Navigation also could reduce the risk of vascular or visceral complications, although studies investigating this have yet to be published.

CONTRAINDICATIONS

Contraindications to the use of a lateral approach are most commonly secondary to conditions that preclude safe or effective lateral access to the lumbar spine. Previous retroperitoneal surgery, such as a nephrectomy, may produce scarring in the retroperitoneal space. Radiation distributed through the approach path, or retroperitoneal infection/abscess history, such as in patients with diverticulitis, are relative contraindications to the lateral approach.[57] Psoas size and position and vascular anatomy may make the approach to L4/5 difficult, and these structures should be scrutinized on cross-sectional imaging as part of the surgical planning process.

COMPLICATIONS

In addition to the known complications of lumbar spine fusion, the lateral approach has unique considerations owing to the approach corridor. These include concern for vascular injuries, lumbar plexus injury, thigh symptoms, ureter injury, hernia, and pseudohernia. Further, the complication profile of ATP and transpsoas techniques vary slightly.

Retroperitoneal incisions and retroperitoneal surgery are known risk factors for pseudohernia. Pseudohernia is a condition in which there is an abdominal wall bulge without violation of the abdominal wall seen in a true hernia. The etiology in the setting of operative trauma is related to denervation of abdominal wall musculature. The pseudohernia rate has been cited in literature at

1.8%; however, much of the literature on this topic fails to distinguish pseudohernia from incisional hernias, limiting the ability to clarify the rate of this complication.[58] In a series reported by Dakwar and colleagues,[58] most cases of pseudohernia resolved by 6 months postoperatively.

Perhaps the most well-recognized risk of lateral approach lumbar spine surgery is the risk of injury to the lumbosacral plexus. Injury occurs in the abdominal wall, retroperitoneal space, or at the level of the psoas.[59] Multiple anatomic studies have shown that safe corridors for transpsoas surgery are larger at the cephalad lumbar segments compared with the caudal segments.[60–62] This is supported by clinical evidence that the risk for nerve injury after LLIF was greater at caudal levels.[63] Motor injury to the subcostal nerve and iliohypogastric nerve can lead to pseudohernia, as previously described. The most commonly reported nerve injured is the lateral femoral cutaneous nerve, which is most at risk at the L4/5 level. The psoas muscle receives direct innervation from the lumbar plexus and is also at risk. Rates of neurologic injury after LLIF reported in the literature range from 0.7% to 22%, but this considerable variability is likely related to inconsistency in the definition of neurologic injury and distinction from thigh symptoms.[64–67] A more recent study demonstrated an approximately 3.7% incidence of plexus pathology from the lateral approach, but reported that the rate of persistent deficit after 18 months had fallen to 2.3%, illustrating the potential for recovery over time.[63] A recent meta-analysis exploring complications of LLIF found that the transpsoas technique was associated with more frequent neurologic and thigh symptoms compared with the ATP technique.[68]

Thigh symptoms remain a common finding after LLIF procedures. These can include anterior thigh pain, dysesthesias, numbness, or hip flexor weakness. Thigh symptoms are quite common from the lateral approach, and to an extent reflect an expected postoperative finding in most cases. The reported rates in the literature vary from 10% to 60%.[65,67,69–73] Because thigh symptoms remain ill-defined, the true incidence of this phenomena postoperatively remains difficult to quantify. What is clear, however, is that most of these symptoms are limited and resolve within a few weeks postoperatively.

Less common complications of LLIF include urologic and vascular injury. There have been case reports of ureter or renal injury in LLIF procedures independent of approach.[74–77] Prompt recognition of this complication when intraoperative hematuria develops or there is persistent flank pain postoperatively can identify the problem and allow for treatment. Reduced rates of vascular injury in LLIF is one of the advantages of the procedure compared with anterior lumbar interbody fusion. However, there are still reports of vascular injury occurring in both the transpsoas and ATP techniques. These include injury to major blood vessels and to segmental vessels.[77–79] The meta-analysis by Walker and colleagues[68] compared rates of vascular injuries in ATP with transpsoas approaches and found a reported rate of major vessel injury with the ATP approach of 1.8% compared with 0.4% in the transpsoas technique.

SUMMARY

LLIF has gained popularity as a technique for placement of wide interbody devices in the treatment of a variety of lumbar conditions. Utilization of this corridor allows placement of a cage that spans the apophyses and enables the ability to achieve clinically significant indirect decompression and deformity correction. In addition, this corridor allows for an extensive disk preparation or debridement, which is appealing in the treatment of degenerative disk disease, diskitis/osteomyelitis, and neoplastic conditions. This versatility of the LLIF is in part related to the lateral access, which allows preservation of posterior stabilizing ligamentous structures in the spine and in some circumstances avoiding more extensive open instrumentation. As experience grows and the technique further evolves, indications may be expanded beyond current limitations.

REFERENCES

1. McAfee PC, Regan JJ, Peter Geis W, et al. Minimally invasive anterior retroperitoneal approach to the lumbar spine. Emphasis on the lateral BAK. Spine (Phila Pa 1976) 1998. https://doi.org/10.1097/00007632-199807010-00009.
2. Ozgur BM, Aryan HE, Pimenta L, et al. Extreme Lateral Interbody Fusion (XLIF): a novel surgical technique for anterior lumbar interbody fusion. Spine J 2006. https://doi.org/10.1016/j.spinee.2005.08.012.
3. Mayer HM. A new microsurgical technique for minimally invasive anterior lumbar interbody fusion. Spine (Phila Pa 1976) 1997. https://doi.org/10.1097/00007632-199703150-00023.
4. Kepler CK, Sama AA, Huang RC, et al. Indirect foraminal decompression after lateral transpsoas interbody fusion. J Neurosurg Spine 2012. https://doi.org/10.3171/2012.1.spine11528.
5. Elowitz EH, Yanni DS, Chwajol M, et al. Evaluation of indirect decompression of the lumbar spinal canal following minimally invasive lateral transpsoas interbody fusion: radiographic and outcome analysis. Minim Invasive Neurosurg 2011. https://doi.org/10.1055/s-0031-1286334.
6. Oliveira L, Marchi L, Coutinho E, et al. A radiographic assessment of the ability of the extreme lateral interbody fusion procedure to indirectly decompress the neural elements. Spine (Phila Pa 1976) 2010. https://doi.org/10.1097/BRS.0b013e3182022db0.
7. Watkins RG, Hanna R, Chang D. Sagittal alignment after lumbar interbody fusion: comparing anterior, lateral, and transforaminal approaches. J Spinal Disord Tech 2014. https://doi.org/10.1097/BSD.0b013e31828a8447.
8. Wang JC, Bohlman HH, Riew KD. Dural tears secondary to operations on the lumbar spine. Management and results after a two-year-minimum follow-up of eighty-eight patients. J Bone Joint Surg Am 1998;80(12):1728–32.
9. Theologis AA, Mundis GM, Nguyen S, et al. Utility of multilevel lateral interbody fusion of the thoracolumbar coronal curve apex in adult deformity surgery in combination with open posterior instrumentation and L5–S1 interbody fusion: a case-matched evaluation of 32 patients. J Neurosurg Spine 2016. https://doi.org/10.3171/2016.8.spine151543.
10. Acosta FL, Liu J, Slimack N, et al. Changes in coronal and sagittal plane alignment following minimally invasive direct lateral interbody fusion for the treatment of degenerative lumbar disease in adults: a radiographic study. J Neurosurg Spine 2011. https://doi.org/10.3171/2011.3.spine10425.
11. Haque RM, Mundis GM, Ahmed Y, et al. Comparison of radiographic results after minimally invasive, hybrid, and open surgery for adult spinal deformity: a multicenter study of 184 patients. Neurosurg Focus 2014. https://doi.org/10.3171/2014.3.focus1424.
12. Daubs MD, Lenke LG, Cheh G, et al. Adult spinal deformity surgery: complications and outcomes in patients over age 60. Spine (Phila Pa 1976) 2007. https://doi.org/10.1097/BRS.0b013e31814cf24a.
13. Uribe JS, Deukmedjian AR, Mummaneni PV, et al. Complications in adult spinal deformity surgery: an analysis of minimally invasive, hybrid, and open surgical techniques. Neurosurg Focus 2014. https://doi.org/10.3171/2014.3.focus13534.
14. Strom RG, Bae J, Mizutani J, et al. Lateral interbody fusion combined with open posterior surgery for adult spinal deformity. J Neurosurg Spine 2016. https://doi.org/10.3171/2016.4.SPINE16157.

15. Park HY, Ha KY, Kim YH, et al. Minimally invasive lateral lumbar interbody fusion for adult spinal deformity. Spine (Phila Pa 1976) 2018. https://doi.org/10.1097/BRS.0000000000002507.

16. Kim KT, Jo DJ, Lee SH, et al. Oblique retroperitoneal approach for lumbar interbody fusion from L1 to S1 in adult spinal deformity. Neurosurg Rev 2018. https://doi.org/10.1007/s10143-017-0927-8.

17. Akbarnia BA, Mundis GM, Moazzaz P, et al. Anterior Column Realignment (ACR) for focal kyphotic spinal deformity using a lateral transpsoas approach and all release. J Spinal Disord Tech 2014. https://doi.org/10.1097/BSD.0b013e318287bdc1.

18. Saigal R, Mundis GM, Eastlack R, et al. Anterior column realignment (ACR) in adult sagittal deformity correction. Spine (Phila Pa 1976) 2016. https://doi.org/10.1097/BRS.0000000000001483.

19. Kotwal S, Kawaguchi S, Lebl D, et al. Minimally invasive lateral lumbar interbody fusion: clinical and radiographic outcome at a minimum 2-year follow-up. J Spinal Disord Tech 2015. https://doi.org/10.1097/BSD.0b013e3182706ce7.

20. Sato J, Ohtori S, Orita S, et al. Radiographic evaluation of indirect decompression of mini-open anterior retroperitoneal lumbar interbody fusion: oblique lateral interbody fusion for degenerated lumbar spondylolisthesis. Eur Spine J 2017. https://doi.org/10.1007/s00586-015-4170-0.

21. Campbell PG, Nunley PD, Cavanaugh D, et al. Short-term outcomes of lateral lumbar interbody fusion without decompression for the treatment of symptomatic degenerative spondylolisthesis at L4–5. Neurosurg Focus 2018. https://doi.org/10.3171/2017.10.focus17566.

22. Alimi M, Hofstetter CP, Tsiouris AJ, et al. Extreme lateral interbody fusion for unilateral symptomatic vertical foraminal stenosis. Eur Spine J 2015. https://doi.org/10.1007/s00586-015-3940-z.

23. Pereira EAC, Farwana M, Lam KS. Extreme lateral interbody fusion relieves symptoms of spinal stenosis and low-grade spondylolisthesis by indirect decompression in complex patients. J Clin Neurosci 2017. https://doi.org/10.1016/j.jocn.2016.09.010.

24. Aichmair A, Alimi M, Hughes AP, et al. Single-level lateral lumbar interbody fusion for the treatment of adjacent segment disease. Spine (Phila Pa 1976) 2017. https://doi.org/10.1097/BRS.0000000000001871.

25. Xu DS, Bach K, Uribe JS. Minimally invasive anterior and lateral transpsoas approaches for closed reduction of grade II spondylolisthesis: initial clinical and radiographic experience. Neurosurg Focus 2018. https://doi.org/10.3171/2017.10.focus17574.

26. Park P, Garton HJ, Gala VC, et al. Adjacent segment disease after lumbar or lumbosacral fusion: review of the literature. Spine (Phila Pa 1976) 2004. https://doi.org/10.1097/01.brs.0000137069.88904.03.

27. Cheh G, Bridwell KH, Lenke LG, et al. Adjacent segment disease followinglumbar/thoracolumbar fusion with pedicle screw instrumentation: a minimum 5-year follow-up. Spine (Phila Pa 1976) 2007. https://doi.org/10.1097/BRS.0b013e31814b2d8e.

28. Radcliff KE, Kepler CK, Jakoi A, et al. Adjacent segment disease in the lumbar spine following different treatment interventions. Spine J 2013. https://doi.org/10.1016/j.spinee.2013.03.020.

29. Palejwala SK, Sheen WA, Walter CM, et al. Minimally invasive lateral transpsoas interbody fusion using a stand-alone construct for the treatment of adjacent segment disease of the lumbar spine: review of the literature and report of three cases. Clin Neurol Neurosurg 2014. https://doi.org/10.1016/j.clineuro.2014.06.031.

30. Louie PK, Varthi AG, Narain AS, et al. Stand-alone lateral lumbar interbody fusion for the treatment of symptomatic adjacent segment degeneration following previous lumbar fusion. Spine J 2018. https://doi.org/10.1016/j.spinee.2018.04.008.

31. Madhavan K, Vanni S, Williams SK. Direct lateral retroperitoneal approach for the surgical treatment of lumbar discitis and osteomyelitis. Neurosurg Focus 2014. https://doi.org/10.3171/2014.6.focus14150.

32. Blizzard DJ, Hills CP, Isaacs RE, et al. Extreme lateral interbody fusion with posterior instrumentation for spondylodiscitis. J Clin Neurosci 2015. https://doi.org/10.1016/j.jocn.2015.05.021.

33. Shepard M, Safain M, Burke SM, et al. Lateral retroperitoneal transpsoas approach to the lumbar spine for the treatment of spondylodiscitis. Minim Invasive Ther Allied Technol 2014. https://doi.org/10.3109/13645706.2014.908924.

34. Karikari IO, Grossi PM, Nimjee SM, et al. Minimally invasive lumbar interbody fusion in patients older than 70 years of age: analysis of peri-and postoperative complications. Neurosurgery 2011. https://doi.org/10.1227/NEU.0b013e3182098bfa.

35. Youssef JA, McAfee PC, Patty CA, et al. Minimally invasive surgery: lateral approach interbody fusion: Results and review. Spine (Phila Pa 1976) 2010. https://doi.org/10.1097/BRS.0b013e3182023438.

36. Smith WD, Dakwar E, Le TV, et al. Minimally invasive surgery for traumatic spinal pathologies: a mini-open, lateral approach in the thoracic and lumbar spine. Spine (Phila Pa 1976) 2010. https://doi.org/10.1097/BRS.0b013e3182023113.

37. Gandhoke GS, Tempel ZJ, Bonfield CM, et al. Technical nuances of the minimally invasive extreme lateral approach to treat thoracolumbar burst fractures. Eur Spine J 2015. https://doi.org/10.1007/s00586-015-3880-7.

38. Theologis AA, Tabaraee E, Toogood P, et al. Anterior corpectomy via the mini-open, extreme lateral, transpsoas approach combined with short-segment posterior fixation for single-level traumatic lumbar burst fractures: analysis of health-related quality of life outcomes and patient satisfaction. J Neurosurg Spine 2015. https://doi.org/10.3171/2015.4.spine14944.

39. Malham GM, Ellis NJ, Parker RM, et al. Maintenance of segmental lordosis and disk height in stand-alone and instrumented extreme lateral interbody fusion (XLIF). Clin Spine Surg 2017. https://doi.org/10.1097/BSD.0b013e3182aa4c94.

40. Marchi L, Abdala N, Oliveira L, et al. Radiographic and clinical evaluation of cage subsidence after stand-alone lateral interbody fusion. J Neurosurg Spine 2013. https://doi.org/10.3171/2013.4.SPINE12319.

41. Kretzer RM, Molina C, Hu N, et al. A comparative biomechanical analysis of stand alone versus facet screw and pedicle screw augmented lateral interbody arthrodesis. Clin Spine Surg 2013. https://doi.org/10.1097/bsd.0b013e3182868ef9.

42. Laws CJ, Coughlin DG, Lotz JC, et al. Direct lateral approach to lumbar fusion is a biomechanically equivalent alternative to the anterior approach: an in vitro study. Spine (Phila Pa 1976) 2012. https://doi.org/10.1097/BRS.0b013e31823551aa.

43. Ahmadian A, Bach K, Bolinger B, et al. Stand-alone minimally invasive lateral lumbar interbody fusion: Multicenter clinical outcomes. J Clin Neurosci 2015. https://doi.org/10.1016/j.jocn.2014.08.036.

44. Williams SK. Indirect decompression for lumbar spinal stenosis with the minimally invasive lateral approach. Semin Spine Surg 2013. https://doi.org/10.1053/j.semss.2013.04.003.

45. Voyadzis J-M, Felbaum D, Rhee J. The rising psoas sign: an analysis of preoperative imaging characteristics of aborted minimally invasive lateral interbody fusions at L4–5. J Neurosurg Spine 2014. https://doi.org/10.3171/2014.1.spine13153.

46. Verla T, Adogwa O, Elsamadicy A, et al. Effects of psoas muscle thickness on outcomes of lumbar fusion surgery. World Neurosurg 2016. https://doi.org/10.1016/j.wneu.2015.11.022.

47. Tohmeh AG, Rodgers WB, Peterson MD. Dynamically evoked, discrete-threshold electromyography in the extreme lateral interbody fusion approach. J Neurosurg Spine 2010. https://doi.org/10.3171/2010.9.spine09871.

48. Krieg SM, Bobinski L, Albers L, et al. Lateral lumbar interbody fusion without intraoperative neuromonitoring: a single-center consecutive series of 157 surgeries. J Neurosurg Spine 2019. https://doi.org/10.3171/2018.9.spine18588.

49. Voyadzis JM, Anaizi AN. Minimally invasive lumbar transfacet screw fixation in the lateral decubitus position after extreme lateral interbody fusion: a technique and feasibility study. J Spinal Disord Tech 2013. https://doi.org/10.1097/BSD.0b013e318241f6c3.

50. Blizzard DJ, Thomas JA. MIS single-position lateral and oblique lateral lumbar interbody fusion and bilateral pedicle screw fixation. Spine (Phila Pa 1976) 2018. https://doi.org/10.1097/BRS.0000000000002330.

51. Ziino C, Konopka JA, Ajiboye RM, et al. Single position versus lateral-then-prone positioning for lateral interbody fusion and pedicle screw fixation. J Spine Surg 2018. https://doi.org/10.21037/jss.2018.12.03.

52. Walker CT, Godzik J, Xu DS, et al. Minimally invasive single-position lateral interbody fusion with robotic bilateral percutaneous pedicle screw fixation: 2-dimensional operative video. Oper Neurosurg (Hagerstown) 2018. https://doi.org/10.1093/ons/opy240.

53. Drazin D, Liu JC, Acosta FL. CT navigated lateral interbody fusion. J Clin Neurosci 2013. https://doi.org/10.1016/j.jocn.2012.12.028.

54. Park P. Three-dimensional computed tomography-based spinal navigation in minimally invasive lateral lumbar interbody fusion: feasibility, technique, and initial results. Neurosurgery 2015. https://doi.org/10.1227/NEU.0000000000000726.

55. Joseph JR, Smith BW, Patel RD, et al. Use of 3D CT-based navigation in minimally invasive lateral lumbar interbody fusion. J Neurosurg Spine 2016. https://doi.org/10.3171/2016.2.spine151295.

56. Zhang YH, White I, Potts E, et al. Comparison perioperative factors during minimally invasive pre-psoas lateral interbody fusion of the lumbar spine using either navigation or conventional fluoroscopy. Global Spine J 2017. https://doi.org/10.1177/2192568217716149.

57. Mobbs R, Phan K, Malham G, et al. Lumbar interbody fusion: techniques, indications and comparison of interbody fusion options including PLIF, TLIF, MI-TLIF, OLIF/ATP, LLIF and ALIF. J Spine Surg 2015. https://doi.org/10.3978/j.issn.2414-469X.2015.10.05.

58. Dakwar E, Le TV, Baaj AA, et al. Abdominal wall paresis as a complication of minimally invasive lateral transpsoas interbody fusion. Neurosurg Focus 2011. https://doi.org/10.3171/2011.7.focus11164.

59. Regev GJ, Kim CW. Safety and the anatomy of the retroperitoneal lateral corridor with respect to the minimally invasive lateral lumbar intervertebral fusion approach. Neurosurg Clin N Am 2014. https://doi.org/10.1016/j.nec.2013.12.001.

60. Benglis DM, Vanni S, Levi AD. An anatomical study of the lumbosacral plexus as related to the minimally invasive transpsoas approach to the lumbar spine.

J Neurosurg Spine 2009. https://doi.org/10.3171/2008.10.spi08479.

61. Park DK, Lee MJ, Lin EL, et al. The relationship of intrapsoas nerves during a transpsoas approach to the lumbar spine: anatomic study. J Spinal Disord Tech 2010. https://doi.org/10.1097/BSD.0b013e3181a9d540.

62. Regev GJ, Chen L, Dhawan M, et al. Morphometric analysis of the ventral nerve roots and retroperitoneal vessels with respect to the minimally invasive lateral approach in normal and deformed spines. Spine (Phila Pa 1976) 2009. https://doi.org/10.1097/BRS.0b013e3181a029e1.

63. Lykissas MG, Aichmair A, Hughes AP, et al. Nerve injury after lateral lumbar interbody fusion: a review of 919 treated levels with identification of risk factors. Spine J 2014. https://doi.org/10.1016/j.spinee.2013.06.066.

64. Sofianos DA, Briseño MR, Abrams J, et al. Complications of the lateral transpsoas approach for lumbar interbody arthrodesis: a case series and literature review. Clin Orthop Relat Res 2012. https://doi.org/10.1007/s11999-011-2088-3.

65. Isaacs RE, Hyde J, Goodrich JA, et al. A prospective, nonrandomized, multicenter evaluation of extreme lateral interbody fusion for the treatment of adult degenerative scoliosis: perioperative outcomes and complications. Spine (Phila Pa 1976) 2010. https://doi.org/10.1097/BRS.0b013e3182022e04.

66. Rodgers WB, Gerber EJ, Patterson J. Intraoperative and early postoperative complications in extreme lateral interbody fusion: an analysis of 600 cases. Spine (Phila Pa 1976) 2011. https://doi.org/10.1097/BRS.0b013e3181e1040a.

67. Pumberger M, Hughes AP, Huang RR, et al. Neurologic deficit following lateral lumbar interbody fusion. Eur Spine J 2012. https://doi.org/10.1007/s00586-011-2087-9.

68. Walker CT, Farber SH, Cole TS, et al. Complications for minimally invasive lateral interbody arthrodesis: a systematic review and meta-analysis comparing prepsoas and transpsoas approaches. J Neurosurg Spine 2019. https://doi.org/10.3171/2018.9.spine18800.

69. Anand N, Rosemann R, Khalsa B, et al. Mid-term to long-term clinical and functional outcomes of minimally invasive correction and fusion for adults with scoliosis. Neurosurg Focus 2010. https://doi.org/10.3171/2010.1.focus09272.

70. Berjano P, Lamartina C. Far lateral approaches (XLIF) in adult scoliosis. Eur Spine J 2013. https://doi.org/10.1007/s00586-012-2426-5.

71. Knight RQ, Schwaegler P, Hanscom D, et al. Direct lateral lumbar interbody fusion for degenerative conditions: Early complication profile. J Spinal Disord Tech 2009. https://doi.org/10.1097/BSD.0b013e3181679b8a.

72. Moller DJ, Slimack NP, Acosta FL, et al. Minimally invasive lateral lumbar interbody fusion and transpsoas approach–related morbidity. Neurosurg Focus 2011. https://doi.org/10.3171/2011.7.FOCUS11137.

73. Cummock MD, Vanni S, Levi AD, et al. An analysis of postoperative thigh symptoms after minimally invasive transpsoas lumbar interbody fusion. J Neurosurg Spine 2011. https://doi.org/10.3171/2011.2.spine10374.

74. Lee HJ, Kim JS, Ryu KS, et al. Ureter injury as a complication of oblique lumbar interbody fusion. World Neurosurg 2017. https://doi.org/10.1016/j.wneu.2017.04.038.

75. Anand N, Baron EM. Urological injury as a complication of the transpsoas approach for discectomy and interbody fusion. J Neurosurg Spine 2012. https://doi.org/10.3171/2012.9.spine12659.

76. Bjurlin MA, Rousseau LA, Vidal PP, et al. Iatrogenic ureteral injury secondary to a thoracolumbar lateral revision instrumentation and fusion. Spine J 2009. https://doi.org/10.1016/j.spinee.2008.12.009.

77. Abe K, Orita S, Mannoji C, et al. Perioperative complications in 155 patients who underwent oblique lateral interbody fusion surgery perspectives and indications from a retrospective, multicenter survey. Spine (Phila Pa 1976) 2017. https://doi.org/10.1097/BRS.0000000000001650.

78. Aichmair A, Fantini GA, Garvin S, et al. Aortic perforation during lateral lumbar interbody fusion. J Spinal Disord Tech 2015. https://doi.org/10.1097/BSD.0000000000000067.

79. Phan K, Maharaj M, Assem Y, et al. Review of early clinical results and complications associated with oblique lumbar interbody fusion (OLIF). J Clin Neurosci 2016. https://doi.org/10.1016/j.jocn.2016.02.030.

Retropleural Thoracic Approach

Joshua T. Wewel, MD[a], Juan S. Uribe, MD[b],*

KEYWORDS

- Thoracic herniated disc • Thoracic discectomy • Retropleural approach
- Minimally invasive surgery

KEY POINTS

- Minimally invasive retropleural technique to thoracic spine is a safe and effective approach for ventral thoracic pathology.
- Patient positioning, incision planning, and access to the thoracic cavity between the endothoracic fascia and parietal pleura are critical steps for a successful surgery.
- Stepwise removal of the rib head, pedicle, ligamentum flavum, developing a partial corpectomy cavity, posterior longitudinal ligament, removal of the disc fragment are the basic steps.

INTRODUCTION

Approaches to the ventral thoracic spine were traditionally posterior in nature. Laminectomy alone carries a high-risk profile with morbidity rates of up to 75%.[1–3] The thoracic spinal cord that is under ventral compression has little reserve for manipulation when attempting to gain access from a posterior, laminectomy-only approach. Additional posterior approaches include the transpedicular, costotransversectomy, and lateral extracavitary approaches. Anterior and lateral approaches subsequently evolved. An anterior transpleural thoracotomy affords often uninhibited access to the ventral thoracic spine and, most important, obviates the need for retraction of the neural elements. However, the anterior thoracotomy carries a longer hospital stay and up to a 27% major complication rate.[4]

More recently, the lateral retropleural thoracic approach has been developed and become more widely used to address the ventral thoracic spine (eg, thoracic disc herniations).[5–10] The lateral retropleural approach offers a minimally invasive alternative for accessing the lateral thoracic spine via a tubular approach. The minimally invasive retropleural approach affords the contemporary surgeon the ability to operate in the extrapleural space, in a familiar tubular environment, and adequately decompress the ventral neural structures without spinal cord manipulation.

INDICATIONS

Patients with radicular pain or myelopathy secondary to ventral thoracic pathology that are recalcitrant to conservative measures are candidates for the retropleural thoracic approach.

CONTRAINDICATIONS

Relative contraindications include previous thoracic surgery, particularly on the side of the desired approach. The intended plane for dissection is between the parietal pleura and endothoracic fascia. If this plane is scarred from previous manipulation, it may drive the dissection intrapleural. The anesthesia advantage of staying within the

Disclosure Statement: J.S. Uribe receives stock options and research support from NuVasive, Inc. Additionally, Dr J.S. Uribe acts as a consultant for Misonix, SI-Bone, and NuVasive, Inc. J.T. Wewel has nothing to disclose.
[a] Department of Neurosurgery, Barrow Neurological Institute, St. Joseph's Hospital and Medical Center, 2910 North 3rd Avenue, Phoenix, AZ 85013, USA; [b] Division of Spinal Disorders, Department of Neurosurgery, Barrow Neurological Institute, St. Joseph's Hospital and Medical Center, 2910 North 3rd Avenue, Phoenix, AZ 85013, USA
* Corresponding author.
E-mail address: Juan.Uribe@barrowbrainandspine.com

Neurosurg Clin N Am 31 (2020) 43–48
https://doi.org/10.1016/j.nec.2019.08.005

plane between the endothoracic fascia and parietal pleura is that single lung ventilation is not needed. Also, an approach surgeon is not needed nor is a postoperative chest tube.

Scoliosis, particularly in the coronal plane, can be a relative or absolute contraindication depending on the severity of the deformity and access to the index disc space. Aberrant vascular anatomy with laterally displaced aorta or inferior vena cava are absolute contraindications.

PREOPERATIVE PLANNING

Preoperative screening requires MRI or a computed tomography (CT) myelogram. MRI and CT scanning allow for a better understanding of the extent of effacement of the thecal sac and compression of the neural elements. Noncontrast CT imaging is also necessary to determine if the herniated disc component is soft or contains some degree of calcified fragments. Additionally, CT imaging provides knowledge of bone anatomy, particularly the vertebral body, pedicles, and the ability to count ribs.

Standing anteroposterior (AP) long cassette radiographs are obtained routinely to study sagittal and coronal balance that may affect surgical planning and counting lumbar vertebra and 12 rib-bearing thoracic vertebra. In cases of obese patients or aberrant anatomy that may contribute to difficulty with intraoperative localization of the index level, a preoperative fiducial can be placed in the pedicle or rib head by interventional radiology. Standard medical clearance is also obtained.

PATIENT POSITIONING

After induction under general anesthesia and intubation, the patient is positioned on a standard, radiolucent operating room table in lateral decubitus position with the intended side of approach facing up. The patient is positioned with the level of the thoracic disc slightly above the break of the table. An axillary role is placed to offset pressure on the brachial plexus and an optional lumbar role is placed above the iliac crest (at the level of the table break) to promote lateral flexion of the trunk and open the intercostal space.

Intraoperative imaging of the surgeon's discretion is then used to localize the index level. Fluoroscopy (with or without computer-assisted stitching software) can be used to count cephalad starting at the sacrum. Alternatively, intraoperative CT scans can be used to assist with localization. The operative table is then positioned such that perfectly orthogonal AP and lateral fluoroscopic images are obtained with the index disc level

parallel to the floor. Neuromonitoring is used in every case with both motor evoked potentials and somatosensory evoked potentials. For high-grade compression, prepositioning and postpositioning signals are monitored.

INCISION PLANNING

When the patient is secured to the operative table and orthogonal radiographs are obtained, the incision is planned. Using lateral fluoroscopy, the projection of the disc space is drawn on the skin. The incision is marked 4 to 6 cm in length, parallel to the traversing rib, ideally passing through the center of the previously drawn projected disc space. The posterior margin of the incision extends slightly posterior to the projected extent of the disc space. For a single-level discectomy, the surgeon can generally plan to resect a portion of only one rib. If the retropleural approach is used for a larger lesion (ie, corpectomy, tumor resection) then 2 partial rib resections may be necessary.

SURGICAL TECHNIQUE

This section describes the technique for a thoracic discectomy. If a corpectomy is planned, the dissection described would have to be expanded to allow vertebral body resection, segmental artery ligation, and hardware placement.

The surgeon stands on the dorsal aspect of the laterally positioned patient. The skin is incised directly superficial and parallel to the previously marked underlying rib. Using monopolar cautery, the soft tissue dissection is carried down until the rib is encountered. The rib is then circumferentially dissected in a subperiosteal manner using a combination of Penfield one, rib dissectors, and Cobb elevators. It is important to carry the rib dissection further than the incision (effectively undermining the incision), particularly posteriorly. Rib resection is carried out with a rib cutter and can be further extended with a rongeur, freeing it from the intercostal muscles, neurovascular bundle and pleura. The posterior remaining remnant rib will limit perpendicular retractor placement at the disc space and should be performed aggressively. The rib is saved for autograft placement.

Once the rib is removed, the intercostal muscles are exposed. Progressive muscle splitting techniques through the muscle exposes the endothoracic fascia and parietal pleura (**Fig. 1**). The endothoracic fascia is often a very fine layer between the muscle and relatively thick parietal pleura. Establishing this plane is key. The natural plane between the endothoracic fascia and parietal pleura develops a potential space (**Fig. 2**). The

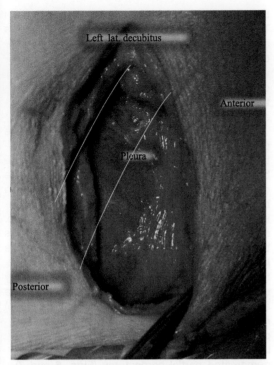

Fig. 1. Cadaveric exposure in the lateral (lat.) decubitus position. Pictured is a dissection after resection of the traversing the targeted rib superior to the targeted disc space. The borders of the dissected rib are highlighted by white lines. Immediately inferior to the resected rib is the pleura.

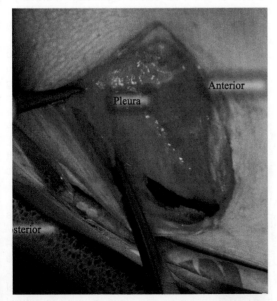

Fig. 2. Further dissection reveals the natural plane that is the retropleural space between the parietal pleura and endothoracic fascia.

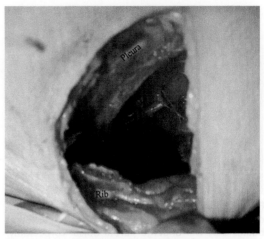

Fig. 3. A minimally invasive, natural, retropleural plane exists and can be developed dorsally and medially. At this point the surgeon must preemptively realize that aggressive dorsal rib resection is important to obtain orthogonal retractor placement. In addition to initial rib resection, piecemeal rongeur resection of residual dorsal rib should be performed.

dissection is carried posteriorly and medially using either digital dissection or blunt instruments and hand-held lung retractor to gently reflect the lung and parietal pleura anterior, effectively separating it from the endothoracic fascia and chest wall. Continued medial exposure reveals the rib head as its costovertebral attachment to the vertebral body, just inferior to the index disc space (**Fig. 3**). Dilators followed by a split blade, expandable retractor can then be placed and connected to a table-mounted attachment (**Fig. 4**). An

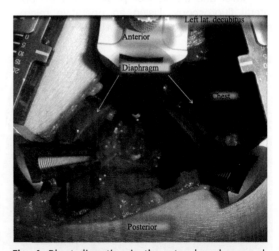

Fig. 4. Blunt dissection in the retropleural space allows for docking of a table-mounted retractor. When attempting dissection at the lower thoracic levels the diaphragm is encountered and can be retracted anterior and inferior. lat., lateral.

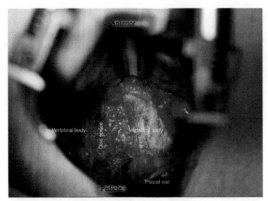

Fig. 5. Final docking of the retractor and further dissection provides visualization of the vertebral bodies that will undergo partial dorsal corpectomy. The pedicle of the inferior vertebra is exposed and will be resected with a high-speed burr until the ligamentum flavum and subsequently lateral thecal sac are exposed.

operative microscope is brought into the field and used for the entirety of the case.

The first bony resection is that of the rib head that can be drilled away with a high-speed burr. When the rib head is removed, the surgeon visualizes the remnant costovertebral joint superficial to the pedicle of the vertebra inferior to the index disc space (**Fig. 5**). The superior margin of the operative field is the pedicle of the vertebral body superior to the disc space and the associated rib head. The posterior margin is the transverse process of the inferior vertebra and the anterior margin is the midpoint of the vertebra.

The next step is to identify and confirm the index disc level and the inferior pedicle with AP and lateral fluoroscopy. Using an operative microscope, the pedicle is drilled with a high-speed

burr, drilling medially toward the spinal canal. The surgeon traverses the cortical, cancellous, and then cortical bone. Intermittent AP fluoroscopy is used to confirm the depth of the drill burr when removing the pedicle. After removing the cortical bone, the ligamentum flavum is encountered and resected with Kerrison rongeurs above and below the disc level.

After ligamentum flavum resection, a partial corpectomy of the superior and inferior vertebral bodies if a discectomy is being performed. The borders of partial corpectomy includes 1 to 2 cm of the inferior portion of the superior vertebral body and 1 to 2 cm of the superior portion of the inferior vertebral body. The AP depth of the partial corpectomy is the dorsal one-third of the vertebral body. The depth of the corpectomy is the contralateral pedicle that can be assessed with intermittent AP fluoroscopy. A high-speed burr can be used for the corpectomy or an ultrasonic blade, easily making linear cuts demarcating the aforementioned borders. When the borders of the corpectomy have been appropriately identified, a large diamond drill bit is then used to remove the demarcated partial corpectomy (**Figs. 6** and **7**). Again, using intermittent fluoroscopy to confirm the depth of drilling. The disc space can be removed with a combination of pituitary and Leksell rongeurs. Posteriorly, the vertebral body is removed until the posterior longitudinal ligament (PLL) is encountered.

Attention is then placed on PLL resection superior and inferior to the disc space. Resecting this portion of the PLL caries significant morbidity because the disc fragment is attached to the PLL at the level of the disc space. Extreme movements can cause dorsal movement of the disc fragment and cause a spinal cord injury. Dorsal maneuvers

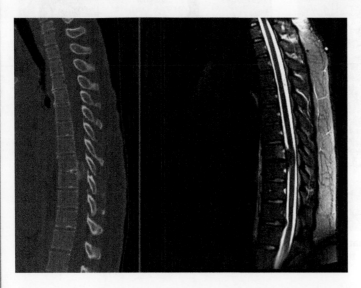

Fig. 6. Noncontrast sagittal CT imaging (*left*) and MRI (*right*) of a preoperative T8 to T9 herniated disc in a 46-year-old man. CT imaging revealed a partially calcified thoracic herniated disc.

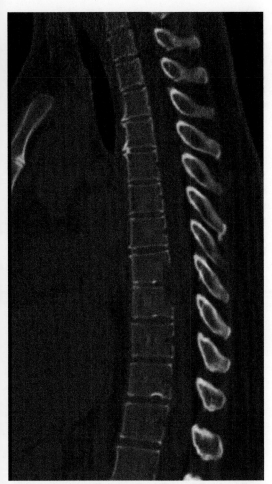

Fig. 7. Postoperative noncontrast, sagittal CT imaging status post minimally invasive retropleural discectomy. Illustrated are the partial corpectomies. The well-defined edges of the corpectomy are achieved with an ultrasonic blade.

in the direction of the cord should be used judiciously. Conversely, aggressive ventral maneuvers should be minimized for fear of rebound of the PLL–disc complex. Use a sharp curette and in a posterior to anterior maneuver to create holes or defects in the PLL. Then, with the use of a Kerrison rongeur, engaging in the previously made PLL defects, the PLL can be resected in a piecemeal manner.

When the PLL has been removed, it will leave behind the remnant PLL–disc complex. A plane is found between the disc and dura, and the disc is pushed ventrally into the previously made corpectomy cavity. Again, anterior maneuvers of the disc fragment without complete release of the fragment can rebound posteriorly and injure the spinal cord. If there are severe adhesions between the disc and dura or there has been dural penetration of the disc through the dura, the disc can be left attached to the dura, floating in the corpectomy cavity after it has been circumferentially dissected from the PLL and vertebral bodies. Meticulous hemostasis is then obtained and the retractor is removed.

CLOSURE

As the retractor is withdrawn, close attention must be paid to the parietal pleura to inspect it for violations. Small violations can be primarily repaired with resorbable sutures. A drain is placed in the retropleural spaced and tunneled subcutaneously. Significant pleural violations may necessitate the placement of a chest tube. The intercostal fascia and musculature are approximated with interrupted absorbable sutures followed by the skin. The drain is water sealed by submerging the tip of the drain underwater and asking the anesthesiologist to perform several Valsalva maneuvers. This step allows the air to be evacuated from the retropleural space and the lung to expand. The drain tubing is clamped, applied to an external suction device, then finally unclamped. Pleural effusion and hemothorax each carry an incidence 1.3% as reported by Baaj and colleagues.[5]

POSTOPERATIVE CARE

After extubation, an AP chest radiograph is obtained immediately in the postanesthesia care unit to rule out a pneumothorax. Typically, these patients are observed in the intensive care unit overnight and mobilized as tolerated. Permitting preoperative significant myelopathy or motor deficit required postoperative inpatient rehabilitation, patients can be discharged home as early as postoperative day 1. As is routinely performed by the senior surgeon, postoperative MRI and CT scans are performed to confirm adequate decompression of the neural elements and visualize the pedicle resection and partial corpectomy (see **Figs. 6** and **7**).

COMPLICATIONS

As with all spine surgeries, dural breach and cerebrospinal fluid (CSF) leak is a risk (2.5%).[5] All CSF leaks should be repaired primarily and aggressively (if possible) to prevent a CSF–pleural fistula. If a primary repair is not possible, an onlay dural substitute can be used in addition to fibrin glue. Additionally, a lumbar drain can be placed as an adjunct to prevent against a persistent CSF leak.

The morbidity of spinal cord injury exists during multiple steps in the procedure. The purpose of drilling the ipsilateral pedicle is to establish the depth and location of the of spinal cord. During all stages of the partial corpectomy, particularly the dorsal bone work, PLL release and resection of the disc fragment are at risk for spinal cord injury. A chronically compressed thoracic spinal cord has very little reserve for manipulation. Slow, deliberate dissection, particularly around the structures abutting the spinal cord, is of utmost importance.

TIPS AND LESSONS LEARNED

At all costs, ensure the correct level is operated on. The preoperative imaging workup is imperative to count lumbar vertebra and rib-bearing thoracic vertebra. Transitional anatomy at the lumbosacral junction and the presence or absence of 12 rib-bearing thoracic vertebral must be defined before establishing the operative plan.

During exposure and rib resection, the neurovascular bundle must be adequately dissected in a subperiosteal manner. As noted, additional posterior rib resection with a Leksell rongeur should be performed to allow for uninhibited orthogonal retractor placement on the vertebral bodies and disc space. When placing and expanding the retractor, attention must be paid toward not compressing the previously dissected and floating neurovascular bundle against the inferior rib. This can cause postoperative costal pain. If this is the case, additional inferior rib resection may need to be performed.

Perform a generous retropleural dissection above and below the targeted disc level to limit unintended tension or cause a tear in the parietal pleura. This factor is especially important if a more extensive procedure is to be performed (ie, full corpectomy, tumor resection).

The use of an ultrasonic blade is particularly useful for defining and making the partial corpectomy borders and cuts (see **Figs. 6** and **7**). A high-speed, large-course diamond burr is an efficient and safe maneuver for completing the partial dorsal corpectomies of the abutting vertebral bodies. PLL resection should be performed with deliberate and conservative, posterior to anterior maneuvers with efforts to avoid rebound of the disc-PLL complex into the thoracic spinal cord.

Regarding the need for fusion, the senior author previously applied a concurrent posterior pedicle screw instrumentation in all cases. Over the past 7 years, posterior instrumentation has been forgone for the following reason. When the pedicle and medial vertebral body are drilled and excised, the anterior vertebral body and anterior longitudinal ligament remain intact. Also, the posterior interspinous ligament and facet complex remain intact. Two of the 3 support columns remain intact and obviate the need for pedicle screw instrumentation. If an aggressive amount of vertebral body resection is necessary, then s full discectomy and arthrodesis should be performed, followed by lateral interbody graft placement and subsequent pedicle screw instrumentation.

SUMMARY

The lateral retropleural approach for ventral thoracic spine pathology is a safe, minimally invasive approach. The workflow described here, when done in a judicious manner, can afford the patient a successful outcome.

REFERENCES

1. Burke TG, Caputy AJ. Treatment of thoracic disc herniation: evolution toward the minimally invasive thoracoscopic technique. Neurosurg Focus 2000;9:e9.
2. Fessler RG, Sturgill M. Review: complications of surgery for thoracic disc disease. Surg Neurol 1998;49: 609–18.
3. McCormick WE, Will SF, Benzel EC. Surgery for thoracic disc disease. Complication avoidance: overview and management. Neurosurg Focus 2000;9:e13.
4. Kerezoudis P, Rajjoub KR, Goncalves S, et al. Anterior versus posterior approaches for thoracic disc herniation: association with postoperative complications. Clin Neurol Neurosurg 2018;167:17–23.
5. Baaj AA, Dakwar E, Le TV, et al. Complications of the mini-open anterolateral approach to the thoracolumbar spine. J Clin Neurosci 2012;19:1265–7.
6. Berjano P, Garbossa D, Damilano M, et al. Transthoracic lateral retropleural minimally invasive microdiscectomy for T9-T10 disc herniation. Eur Spine J 2014;23:1376–8.
7. Kasliwal MK, Deutsch H. Minimally invasive retropleural approach for central thoracic disc herniation. Minim Invasive Neurosurg 2011;54:167–71.
8. Moran C, Ali Z, McEvoy L, et al. Mini-open retropleural transthoracic approach for the treatment of giant thoracic disc herniation. Spine 2012;37:E1079–84.
9. Uribe JS, Dakwar E, Cardona RF, et al. Minimally invasive lateral retropleural thoracolumbar approach: cadaveric feasibility study and report of 4 clinical cases. Neurosurgery 2011;68:32–9 [discussion: 39].
10. Uribe JS, Smith WD, Pimenta L, et al. Minimally invasive lateral approach for symptomatic thoracic disc herniation: initial multicenter clinical experience. J Neurosurg Spine 2012;16:264–79.

Novel Intervertebral Technologies

Mohamad Bydon, MD[a,b,*], Anshit Goyal, MBBS[a,b], Yagiz U. Yolcu, MD[a,b]

KEYWORDS

- Degenerative spine disease • Intervertebral disk herniation • Intervertebral cages
- Expandable cages • Composite cages • Annuloplasty • 3D printing • Regenerative medicine

KEY POINTS

- Expandable mechanical cages may serve as useful devices for correcting lordosis in patients undergoing spinal fusion.
- Expandable mesh cages provide a feasible alternative for graft delivery, especially in treatment of spinal fractures.
- Modern composite cage designs, such as titanium and polyether ether ketone (PEEK), are commonly used and reported to have fusion rates as high as 96%.
- Annular repair/annuloplasty technologies have emerged as an adjunctive treatment approach to lumbar diskectomy for lumbar disk herniation.
- Future efforts are shifting toward additive manufacturing, such as 3D printing.

INTRODUCTION

Degenerative spine disease is a chronic disorder bearing a significant annual cost in terms of morbidity, lost productivity, and quality-adjusted life years. Surgical procedures, such as spinal fusion and disk replacement, are commonly used for treatment on failure of conservative treatment. However, there is growing consensus that currently available surgical technologies may have long-term inefficacy for successful management. Intervertebral disk degeneration is the most common manifestation of degenerative spine disease; hence, replacement/repair of this tissue is an important component of surgical treatment. At the same time, restoration of spinal alignment and preservation of natural kinematics is essential to a good outcome. This article reviews novel intervertebral implant technologies that may have the potential to significantly impact elective spine surgery for degenerative spine disease.

NOVEL INTERBODY CAGES
Expandable Mechanical Cages

Expandable cages are among novel technologies that are used in spinal fusion procedures. The hypothesized mechanisms for expandable cages are lengthening the anterior column to achieve lordotic correction, and minimizing neural retraction and tissue disruption during cage placement.[1] Although they have been used for more than 10 years now, cages are relatively new considering the history of spinal surgery and specifically, fusion procedures. Moreover, there is an increasing trend in utilization after the introduction of multiple different cages in early 2010s (eg, CALIBER and RISE, Globus Medical, Inc, Audubon, PA).[2] Currently, various types of cages exist, including specific types for different approaches. **Fig. 1** illustrates a schematic for expandable mechanical cages.

Disclosures: The authors have nothing to disclose.
[a] Mayo Clinic Neuro-Informatics Laboratory, Mayo Clinic, Rochester, MN, USA; [b] Department of Neurologic Surgery, Mayo Clinic, Charlton building, Room 6-124, 201 West Center Street, Rochester, MN 55902, USA
* Corresponding author. Department of Neurologic Surgery, Mayo Clinic, Gonda building, 8th floor, 200 1st Street Southwest, Rochester, MN 55905.
E-mail address: bydon.mohamad@mayo.edu

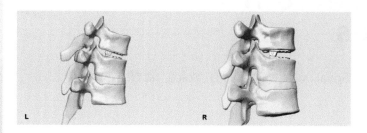

Fig. 1. Expandable mechanical cage (*left*). Lordotic correction on expansion (*right*).

Several studies have investigated the biomechanical properties of expandable cages using cadaveric spine specimens. Transforaminal lumbar interbody fusion (TLIF) with expandable cages reduced flexion-extension motion significantly.[3] When tested for lateral bending motion, expandable cages were also found to limit the motion significantly.[3] When tested in single segment posterior lumbar interbody fusion, similar results were obtained with TLIF experiments; however, a need for the addition of pedicle screws was also noted.[4] Radiographic outcomes for the use of expandable cages were assessed by carrying out comparisons with nonexpandable alternatives. An analysis of 89 patients by Yee and colleagues[1] revealed lower segmental lordosis (2° vs 3° at 1 month; 1° vs 3° at 1 year) and higher lumbar lordosis (2° vs 1° at 1 month; 5° vs 2° at 1 year) in expandable group with differences being statistically nonsignificant.

Moreover, a recent meta-analysis comparing clinical and radiographic outcomes between expandable and nonexpandable cages assessed the increase in disk height, the change in lumbar lordosis, and segmental lordosis at the last follow-up.[5] Mean increase in disk height was found to be significantly higher in studies using nonexpandable cages, whereas segmental lordosis was significantly higher for expandable cages. Lumbar lordosis and secondary outcome measures, such as fusion rate, reoperations, and subsidence rates, did not differ between two groups.[5]

Although less common than the lumbar spine, expandable cages are also used in cervical spine procedures. However, so far, only level IV evidence in the form of case reports, case series, or small retrospective studies has been reported in the literature.[6–8] They are currently being used for a broad range of conditions including degenerative diseases, tumors, or deformity cases.[9] A systematic review of the literature by Elder and colleagues[10] summarized 24 studies involving expandable cage use in cervical fusion surgeries. Overall, the authors concluded that expandable cages may be used in patients with low bone quality and they could provide a safe alternative to other methods.[10]

Expandable Mesh Cages

Mesh implants are designed to insert bone grafts in the intervertebral space or defects created by bone injuries. The empty mesh is introduced into the space with the help of a cannula, and then filled with the bone graft.[11] These devices are intended to be used in fractures of thoracolumbar spine, such as osteoporotic compression fractures. Similar to expandable mechanical cages, expandable mesh bags/cages are thought to minimize surrounding soft tissue and nerve injury mainly by reducing the amount of retraction during surgery. Moreover, porous structures are suggested to create an osteoconductive environment for the grafts.

A biomechanical study evaluating Optimesh (Spineology Inc, St. Paul, MN)[11] graft containment system showed similar range of motion parameters in axial torsion, lateral bending, and flexion-extension compared with standard TLIF procedure.[12] An example of the use of this technology was reported in 2006 in a case report, where a 47-year-old male patient with L1 vertebral injury was treated with expandable mesh with posterior fixation of T12-L2.[13] The patient was reportedly pain-free soon following the surgery with correction of the fracture-associated deformity.[13] Another study on a larger cohort using a titanium mesh (OsseoFix, Alphatec Spine Inc, Carlsbad, CA)[14] evaluated clinical and radiologic outcomes for patients with osteoporotic thoracolumbar burst fractures. Significant improvements in Oswestry Disability Index (ODI) and Visual Analogue Scale (VAS) scores were found in addition to improvement in Cobb angle for kyphosis and a low subsidence rate (6.8%).[15]

Literature to date shows promising results from biomechanical studies and small case reports and case series. However, larger evaluations, especially randomized clinical trials, are required to obtain stronger evidence for use of these devices. It is also important to note that use of expandable mesh cages has not been reported in the cervical spine, as opposed to expandable mechanical cages.

Modern Composite Cage Designs

Titanium (Ti) and polyether ether ketone (PEEK) had been the most commonly used materials in development of cages since cages started to be used in spinal fusion surgeries. However, both materials had certain drawbacks when used alone.[16] Ti cages were associated with higher subsidence rates and had limitations in fusion assessment because of lack of radiolucency.[17–19] In contrast, PEEK cages were associated with pseudarthrosis when used alone.[20] Therefore, recent efforts have been directed toward merging two materials in a single device and create more efficacious cages while reducing complications.[21]

Clinical outcomes for Ti/PEEK cages have been recently started to be reported in the literature. A recent study by Chong and colleagues[22] showed a fusion rate of 96%, followed by an analysis of 47 patients undergoing anterior diskectomy and fusion with achievement of 96% fusion rate.[23] Similar results were obtained with regards to lumbar fusion procedures. A randomized clinical trial comparing the use of Ti/PEEK cages with PEEK-only cages among patients undergoing TLIF showed fusion rates greater than 90% at 3-month follow-up.[24] Further, assessment of Ti/PEEK cages in anterior lumbar interbody fusion procedures reported a fusion rate of 95% with significant improvement in VAS and ODI scores at last follow-up.[25]

ANNULOPLASTY TECHNOLOGIES

Lumbar diskectomy is an effective treatment option for radiculopathy caused by intervertebral disk herniation, as demonstrated by randomized controlled studies.[26–28] However, analysis from large administrative databases has shown that up to 18% of lumbar diskectomies may eventually require revision surgery because of recurrent lumbar disk herniation (LDH).[29] It is further postulated that nerve root decompression via diskectomy may weaken the annulus fibrosus, causing consequent dehydration of the nucleus pulposus and loss of disk height, which may cause re-exacerbation of radicular symptoms.[30] Recently, annular repair/annuloplasty technologies have been proposed to counter the incidence of recurrent LDH and disk height loss following lumbar diskectomy. Among them include annular closure devices (ACDs), such as Barricaid (Intrinsic Therapeutics, Inc, Woburn, MA), and an annular tissue repair system (AR)-Annulex-Xclose (Anulex Technologies, Minnetonka, MN).

Barricaid is a bone-anchored ACD that comprises of a Ti anchor portion inserted into the adjacent vertebral body while a polymer mesh portion serves to block the annular defect, thereby reducing the incidence of recurrent LDH.[31–33] **Fig. 2** illustrates a schematic for a bone-anchored ACD. In the past decade, a growing body of clinical studies have evaluated ACDs as an adjunct following lumbar diskectomy.[31–39] ACDs have been shown to confer greater improvement in leg pain as compared with diskectomy alone.[32,34] In a cohort study of 157 subjects (Barricaid-63 vs Control-94), Trummer and colleagues[33] demonstrated a lower rate of facet joint degeneration with use of the Barricaid device. Use of ACD is also suggested to be associated with preservation of disk height.[32] However, the primary objective of using ACDs (a reduction in rate of reherniation) is yet to be demonstrated via level I evidence. In a multicenter prospective cohort study evaluating the Barricaid device, Parker and colleagues[32] demonstrated a lower reherniation rate with annular closure (0% vs 6.5%) after 2 years of follow-up, which was not statistically significant. The study was, however, underpowered to detect differences. In follow-up results from the same study, the investigators projected estimated cost savings of $2226 per diskectomy when done with an ACD, because of reduction of recurrent disk herniation, when modeled on US Medicare costs.[35] In a single arm, prospective clinical trial (75 subjects), Bouma and colleagues[39] showed a symptomatic reherniation rate of 1.5% at 2 years. However, the trial lacked a comparison arm and the results were only compared with reherniation rates reported in the literature (2%–18%). Two-year follow-up results from the largest randomized clinical trial to date are still awaited.[31] In a post hoc analysis from the same trial, the investigators

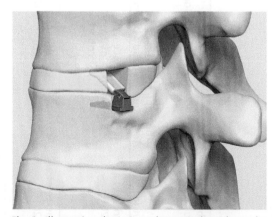

Fig. 2. Illustration depicting a bone-anchored annular closure device.

Table 1
Studies evaluating annular repair technologies

Author, Year	Annuloplasty Technique	Study Design	Patient Population	Comparator	Sample Size (Annuloplasty)	Sample Size (Comparison Group)	Follow-up (mo)	Outcomes Evaluated	Results
Parker et al,[32] 2016	ACD (Barricaid)	P; O; MC, matched cohort	Single-level lumbar diskectomy	Yes; diskectomy alone	30	46	24	VAS, ODI, reherniation	Significant reduction in VAS-LP and ODI at 1 y with ACD, similar reherniation rate
Klassen et al,[31] 2016	ACD (Barricaid)	P; RCT; MC; post hoc ITT analysis	Single-level lumbar diskectomy	Yes; diskectomy alone	272	278	1.5	Complications; reoperations	Significantly lower 90-d complication and reoperation rate with ACD
Klassen et al,[37] 2017	ACD (Barricaid)	P; RCT; MC	Single-level lumbar diskectomy	Yes; diskectomy alone	272	278	1.5	ODI, VAS, SF-36, disk height, reherniation	Results awaited
Vukas et al,[34] 2013	ACD (Barricaid)	P; O; MC	Single-level lumbar diskectomy	Yes; diskectomy alone	30	72	24	VAS, ODI, reherniation	No symptomatic reherniation in either group; significantly lower VAS-LP in ACD group at last follow-up
Parker et al,[35] 2013	ACD (Barricaid)	P; O; MC, matched cohort	Single-level lumbar diskectomy	Yes; diskectomy alone	30	46	24	Cost	Cost savings of $2226 per diskectomy with ACD; modeled on Medicare costs
Lequin et al,[36] 2012	ACD (Barricaid)	P; SA; clinical trial	Limited lumbar diskectomy	No	45	—	12	VAS, ODI, reherniation	1 reherniation (2.4%); significant improvement in VAS and ODI

Trummer et al,[33] 2013	ACD (Barricaid)	P; MC; O	Single-level lumbar diskectomy	Yes; diskectomy alone	63	94	12	VAS, ODI, facet degeneration	Significantly lower incidence of facet degeneration with ACD
Bouma et al,[39] 2013	ACD (Barricaid)	P; SA; clinical trial	Single-level lumbar diskectomy	No	75	—	24	VAS, ODI, reherniation	1 (1.4%) symptomatic reherniation among 73 followed patients; significant improvement in VAS and ODI
Hahn et al,[38] 2014	ACD (Barricaid)	R; O; SA; SC	Single-level lumbar diskectomy	No	3	—	12	VAS, disk height	Reduction in VAS-BP and VAS-LP; preservation of disk height in all 3 cases
Bailey et al,[40] 2013	AR (Annulex-X-close)	P; RCT; MC	1–2 level lumbar diskectomy; baseline VAS-LP >4	Yes; diskectomy alone	478	272	24	VAS, ODI, SF-12, reherniation	Overall, lower but statistically nonsignificant reherniation with use of AR; subgroup analysis of predominant leg pain patients showed statistically significant reduction in reherniation risk; no difference in PROs

Abbreviations: ITT, intention-to-treat; MC, multicenter; NRCT, nonrandomized clinical trial (with comparison); O, observational; P, prospective; PRO, patient-reported outcome; R, retrospective; RCT, randomized controlled trial; SA, single-arm (no comparison); SC, single-center; VAS-BP, visual Analog Scale-Back Pain; VAS-LP, Visual Analog Scale-Leg Pain.

reported significantly lower 90-day reoperation rates (1.9% vs 5.4%) with annular closure compared with diskectomy alone.[37]

The Anulex Xclose tissue repair system comprises of single or multiple tension bands of nonabsorbable suture loop attached to two tissue anchors placed on either side of the annular defect.[30] In contrast to the ACDs, evidence regarding direct annular repair systems is more limited, with only a single study published to date.[40] In a single-blind, randomized controlled trial of 750 patients (500 undergoing lumbar diskectomy with AR, 250 undergoing diskectomy alone), patients undergoing annular repair had lower rates of reherniation versus those that underwent diskectomy alone at all follow-up time points (3 months, 4.5% vs 2.2%; 6 months, 6.2% vs 4.1%; 2 years, 11.2% vs 9.2%); however these differences were not statistically significant in the overall study comparison.[40] Subgroup analysis revealed significant reduction in rate of reherniation (absolute risk reduction: 83% [$P = .02$] and 71% [$P = .04$] at 3-month and 6-month follow-up, respectively) for those subjects presenting with predominant leg pain. In addition, although significant improvements were noted in ODI and Short Form-12 Physical Component Score in either group, no significant difference was noted between groups. Subjects were only enrolled into the trial at the discretion of the treating surgeon if the size of the annular defect was deemed sufficient for reapproximation. These results suggest the need for appropriate patient selection for annular repair in addition to diskectomy. **Table 1** summarizes the studies reporting outcomes following use of annular repair technologies in conjunction with lumbar microdiskectomy.

However, there are notable limitations to the use of annular closure technologies. Large disk extrusions and annular defects would render usage of ACDs unsuitable. For example, the Barricaid device was restricted to be used with annular defects less than 6 mm in height and less than 10 mm in width. Use of the Anulex AR device would also require sufficient disk height and reasonable defect area.[30] Presence of other spinal deformities, such as spondylolisthesis, would also preclude use because of difficult implantation.

PERSONALIZED INTERVERTEBRAL IMPLANTS

The advent of additive manufacturing, commonly known as three-dimensional (3D) printing, has paved rise of the possibility of inexpensive, patient-specific implants for use in spine surgery. Size mismatch is an important challenge to intervertebral cage placement because commercially available implants may not always be specific to patient anatomy. Studies using patient specific 3D-printed intervertebral disk implants have been reported but are currently limited by lack of follow-up data.[41–43] Theoretically, development of such novel anatomically shaped intervertebral cages should allow for higher load transfer, preventing damage to cortical bone and accelerating the fusion process with reduction in implant dislocation.[44–46] In addition, avoidance of size mismatch allows for more efficient surgical planning and shorter operative time. Additional graft material may be packed with the implant.[42] Multiple cases with successful use of such implants have been reported in the cervical spine;[41,42,47] however, published studies on lumbar intervertebral cage implantation are more limited.[42,43]

Regenerative medicine and tissue engineering approaches may be promising sources of novel intervertebral technologies for biologic disk repair/replacement by allowing for 3D printing of interverebral disk tissue in the future.[48,49] Intervertebral disk transplantation has been attempted in animal models[50–52] and more recently in humans.[53] Stem cell implantation into the intervertebral disk has been suggested as a means to reverse/delay degenerative changes in experimental models of disk degeneration.[48] However, replacement using engineered tissue rather than cells may be a more effective means of preserving spinal motion and kinematics. Several sources of stem cells have been suggested to be capable of producing intervertebral disk tissue.[48] However, further work on scaffold selection, cell culture, and navigation of several other in vivo challenges is required for this area to attain the requisite conceptual maturity for regulatory approval and more widespread clinical application.

ACKNOWLEDGMENTS

The authors acknowledge the efforts of James Postier, a medical illustrator at Mayo Clinic in Rochester, Minnesota who created the illustrations used in this article.

REFERENCES

1. Yee TJ, Joseph JR, Terman SW, et al. Expandable vs static cages in transforaminal lumbar interbody fusion: radiographic comparison of segmental and lumbar sagittal angles. Neurosurgery 2017;81(1): 69–74.

2. expandabletechnology – Globus Expandable Technology. Available at: http://globusmedical.com/ expandabletechnology/. Accessed April 29, 2019.

3. Mica MC, Voronov LI, Carandang G, et al. Biomechanics of an expandable lumbar interbody fusion cage deployed through transforaminal approach. Int J Spine Surg 2018;12(4):520–7.

4. Bhatia NN, Lee KH, Bui CN, et al. Biomechanical evaluation of an expandable cage in single-segment posterior lumbar interbody fusion. Spine 2012;37(2):E79–85.

5. Alvi MA, Kurian SJ, Wahood W, et al. Assessing the difference in clinical and radiologic outcomes between expandable cage and nonexpandable cage among patients undergoing minimally invasive transforaminal interbody fusion: a systematic review and meta-analysis. World Neurosurg 2019. https://doi.org/10.1016/j.wneu.2019.03.284.

6. Burkett CJ, Baaj AA, Dakwar E, et al. Use of titanium expandable vertebral cages in cervical corpectomy. J Clin Neurosci 2012;19(3):402–5.

7. Ayhan S, Palaoglu S, Geyik S, et al. Concomitant intramedullary arteriovenous malformation and a vertebral hemangioma of cervical spine discovered by a pathologic fracture during bicycle accident. Eur Spine J 2015;24(1):187–92.

8. Omeis I, Bekelis K, Gregory A, et al. The use of expandable cages in patients undergoing multilevel corpectomies for metastatic tumors in the cervical spine. Orthopedics 2010;33(2):87–92.

9. Zhang HY, Thongtrangan I, Le H, et al. Expandable cage for cervical spine reconstruction. J Korean Neurosurg Soc 2005;38:435–41.

10. Elder BD, Lo SF, Kosztowski TA, et al. A systematic review of the use of expandable cages in the cervical spine. Neurosurg Rev 2016;39(1):1–11 [discussion: 11].

11. OptiMesh Graft Containment | Spineology. Available at: https://www.spineology.com/united-states/our-products/optimesh%C2%AE-graft-containment. Accessed April 29, 2019.

12. Zheng X, Chaudhari R, Wu C, et al. Biomechanical evaluation of an expandable meshed bag augmented with pedicle or facet screws for percutaneous lumbar interbody fusion. Spine J 2010;10(11):987–93.

13. Inamasu J, Guiot BH, Uribe JS. Flexion-distraction injury of the L1 vertebra treated with short-segment posterior fixation and Optimesh. J Clin Neurosci 2008;15(2):214–8.

14. OsseoFix Spinal Fracture Reduction System - Alphatec Spine. Alphatec Spine. Available at: https://atecspine.com/product-portfolio/thoracolumbar/osseofix-spinal-fracture-reduction-system/. Accessed April 29, 2019.

15. Ender SA, Eschler A, Ender M, et al. Fracture care using percutaneously applied titanium mesh cages (OsseoFix) for unstable osteoporotic thoracolumbar burst fractures is able to reduce cement-associated complications: results after 12 months. J Orthop Surg Res 2015. https://doi.org/10.1186/s13018-015-0322-5.

16. McGilvray KC, Waldorff EI, Easley J, et al. Evaluation of a polyetheretherketone (PEEK) titanium composite interbody spacer in an ovine lumbar interbody fusion model: biomechanical, microcomputed tomographic, and histologic analyses. Spine J 2017;17(12):1907–16.

17. Chen Y, Wang X, Lu X, et al. Comparison of titanium and polyetheretherketone (PEEK) cages in the surgical treatment of multilevel cervical spondylotic myelopathy: a prospective, randomized, control study with over 7-year follow-up. Eur Spine J 2013;22(7):1539–46.

18. Niu CC, Liao JC, Chen WJ, et al. Outcomes of interbody fusion cages used in 1 and 2-levels anterior cervical discectomy and fusion: titanium cages versus polyetheretherketone (PEEK) cages. J Spinal Disord Tech 2010;23(5):310–6.

19. Han CM, Lee EJ, Kim HE, et al. The electron beam deposition of titanium on polyetheretherketone (PEEK) and the resulting enhanced biological properties. Biomaterials 2010;31(13):3465–70.

20. Duncan JW, Bailey RA. An analysis of fusion cage migration in unilateral and bilateral fixation with transforaminal lumbar interbody fusion. Eur Spine J 2013;22(2):439–45.

21. Assem Y, Mobbs RJ, Pelletier MH, et al. Radiological and clinical outcomes of novel Ti/PEEK combined spinal fusion cages: a systematic review and preclinical evaluation. Eur Spine J 2017;26(3):593–605.

22. Chong E, Mobbs RJ, Pelletier MH, et al. Titanium/polyetheretherketone cages for cervical arthrodesis with degenerative and traumatic pathologies: early clinical outcomes and fusion rates. Orthop Surg 2016;8(1):19–26.

23. Phan K, Pelletier MH, Rao PJ, et al. Integral fixation titanium/polyetheretherketone cages for cervical arthrodesis: evolution of cage design and early radiological outcomes and fusion rates. Orthop Surg 2019;11(1):52–9.

24. Rickert M, Fleege C, Tarhan T, et al. Transforaminal lumbar interbody fusion using polyetheretherketone oblique cages with and without a titanium coating: a randomised clinical pilot study. Bone Joint J 2017;99-B(10):1366–72.

25. Mobbs RJ, Phan K, Assem Y, et al. Combination Ti/PEEK ALIF cage for anterior lumbar interbody fusion: early clinical and radiological results. J Clin Neurosci 2016;34:94–9.

26. Weinstein JN, Lurie JD, Tosteson TD, et al. Surgical versus nonoperative treatment for lumbar disc herniation: four-year results for the Spine Patient Outcomes Research Trial (SPORT). Spine 2008;33(25):2789–800.

27. Weinstein JN, Lurie JD, Tosteson TD, et al. Surgical vs nonoperative treatment for lumbar disk herniation: the Spine Patient Outcomes Research

Trial (SPORT) observational cohort. JAMA 2006; 296(20):2451–9.

28. Lurie JD, Tosteson TD, Tosteson AN, et al. Surgical versus nonoperative treatment for lumbar disc herniation: eight-year results for the spine patient outcomes research trial. Spine 2014;39(1):3–16.

29. Virk SS, Diwan A, Phillips FM, et al. What is the rate of revision discectomies after primary discectomy on a national scale? Clin Orthop Relat Res 2017; 475(11):2752–62.

30. Choy WJ, Phan K, Diwan AD, et al. Annular closure device for disc herniation: meta-analysis of clinical outcome and complications. BMC Musculoskelet Disord 2018;19(1):290.

31. Klassen PD, Hes R, Bouma GJ, et al. A multicenter, prospective, randomized study protocol to demonstrate the superiority of a bone-anchored prosthesis for anular closure used in conjunction with limited discectomy to limited discectomy alone for primary lumbar disc herniation. Int J Clin Trials 2016;3(3): 120–31.

32. Parker SL, Grahovac G, Vukas D, et al. Effect of an annular closure device (Barricaid) on same-level recurrent disk herniation and disk height loss after primary lumbar discectomy: two-year results of a multicenter prospective cohort study. Clin Spine Surg 2016;29(10):454–60.

33. Trummer M, Eustacchio S, Barth M, et al. Protecting facet joints post-lumbar discectomy: Barricaid annular closure device reduces risk of facet degeneration. Clin Neurol Neurosurg 2013;115(8):1440–5.

34. Vukas D, Ledić D, Grahovac G, et al. Clinical outcomes in patients after lumbar disk surgery with annular reinforcement device: two-year follow up. Acta Clin Croat 2013;52(1):87–91.

35. Parker SL, Grahovac G, Vukas D, et al. Cost savings associated with prevention of recurrent lumbar disc herniation with a novel annular closure device: a multicenter prospective cohort study. J Neurol Surg A Cent Eur Neurosurg 2013;74(5):285–9.

36. Lequin MB, Barth M, Thomé C, et al. Primary limited lumbar discectomy with an annulus closure device: one-year clinical and radiographic results from a prospective, multi-center study. Korean J Spine 2012;9(4):340–7.

37. Klassen PD, Bernstein DT, Köhler HP, et al. Bone-anchored annular closure following lumbar discectomy reduces risk of complications and reoperations within 90 days of discharge. J Pain Res 2017;10: 2047–55.

38. Hahn BS, Ji GY, Moon B, et al. Use of annular closure device (Barricaid) for preventing lumbar disc reherniation: one-year results of three cases. Korean J Neurotrauma 2014;10(2):119–22.

39. Bouma GJ, Barth M, Ledic D, et al. The high-risk discectomy patient: prevention of reherniation in patients with large annular defects using an annular closure device. Eur Spine J 2013;22(5):1030–6.

40. Bailey A, Araghi A, Blumenthal S, et al. Prospective, multicenter, randomized, controlled study of annular repair in lumbar discectomy: two-year follow-up. Spine 2013;38(14):1161–9.

41. Phan K, Sgro A, Maharaj MM, et al. Application of a 3D custom printed patient specific spinal implant for C1/2 arthrodesis. J Spine Surg 2016;2(4):314–8.

42. The utility of 3D printing for surgical planning and patient-specific implant design for complex spinal pathologies: case report. J Neurosurg Spine 2017; 26(4):513–8.

43. Serra T, Capelli C, Toumpaniari R, et al. Design and fabrication of 3D-printed anatomically shaped lumbar cage for intervertebral disc (IVD) degeneration treatment. Biofabrication 2016;8(3):035001.

44. Burton AK, Balagué F, Cardon G, et al. Chapter 2. European guidelines for prevention in low back pain: November 2004. Eur Spine J 2006;15(Suppl 2):S136–68.

45. Malandrino A, Noailly J, Lacroix D. The effect of sustained compression on oxygen metabolic transport in the intervertebral disc decreases with degenerative changes. PLoS Comput Biol 2011;7(8): e1002112.

46. Giorgi H, Prébet R, Delhaye M, et al. Minimally invasive posterior transforaminal lumbar interbody fusion: one-year postoperative morbidity, clinical and radiological results of a prospective multicenter study of 182 cases. Orthop Traumatol Surg Res 2015;101(6 Suppl):S241–5.

47. Spetzger U, Frasca M, König SA. Surgical planning, manufacturing and implantation of an individualized cervical fusion titanium cage using patient-specific data. Eur Spine J 2016;25(7):2239–46.

48. Kandel R, Roberts S, Urban JP. Tissue engineering and the intervertebral disc: the challenges. Eur Spine J 2008;17(Suppl 4):480–91.

49. Cho W, Job AV, Chen J, et al. A review of current clinical applications of three-dimensional printing in spine surgery. Asian Spine J 2018;12(1):171–7.

50. Frick SL, Hanley EN Jr, Meyer RA Jr, et al. Lumbar intervertebral disc transfer. A canine study. Spine 1994;19(16):1826–34 [discussion: 1834–5].

51. Luk KD, Ruan DK, Chow DH, et al. Intervertebral disc autografting in a bipedal animal model. Clin Orthop Relat Res 1997;337:13–26.

52. Olson EJ, Hanley EN Jr, Rudert MJ, et al. Vertebral column allografts for the treatment of segmental spine defects. An experimental investigation in dogs. Spine 1991;16(9):1081–8.

53. Ruan D, He Q, Ding Y, et al. Intervertebral disc transplantation in the treatment of degenerative spine disease: a preliminary study. Lancet 2007; 369(9566):993–9.

Surface Technologies in Spinal Fusion

Jacob J. Enders, BS[a], Daniel Coughlin, MD[b], Thomas E. Mroz, MD[b],*, Shaleen Vira, MD[b]

KEYWORDS

- Lumbar interbody fusion • Surface technology • Modification • Cage

KEY POINTS

- Autograft and allograft bone are traditional surface technologies that enjoy a long documentation of clinical success.
- Novel technologies have been developed that approach but have not surpassed these traditional technologies.
- Polyetheretherketone has been used in spine fusion as an alternative to traditional metal materials to limit stress shielding and improve radiolucency, but has limited bony integration.
- Bioactive ceramics and surface coatings with materials such as titanium have been developed with modest clinical results.
- There is little high-level evidence supporting the various bioengineered cage surface technologies. Additional studies are needed to support their clinical use.

INTRODUCTION

Interbody fusion is often used in addition to decompression to realign displaced vertebral bodies and correct spinal instability.[1,2] This article summarizes the various materials and surface properties that have been developed in the last 3 decades that serve as interbody cage and/or intervertebral spacers that facilitate spinal fusion (**Fig. 1**). Additionally, we describe the original technologies of titanium and polyetheretherketone (PEEK), and then expand into newer surface technologies including bioactive glasses and ceramics, porous titanium, surface modifications to PEEK, and tantalum.

TITANIUM SURFACE TECHNOLOGY

Titanium and its alloys, most notably Ti-6Al-4V, have become common in spinal interbody cages.

One reason for this trend is the ability of titanium to form a nonreactive TiO_2 surface layer and facilitate bone growth in and around the implant.[3] In a 1994 study, Leong and colleagues[4] demonstrated bone growth in 18 of 23 patients receiving titanium mesh blocks as intervertebral disk spacers without the need of an autologous bone graft. More recent work has demonstrated that introducing microscale and nanoscale roughness on the surface of Ti specimens can result in increased osteoblast maturation.[5–7] However, titanium on its own has significant drawbacks, including a high elastic modulus of about 110 GPa that can contribute to stress shielding and implant subsidence.[8–10] Titanium is also radiopaque, making it difficult to determine the extent bony fusion around the implants, while producing significant beam artifact on computed tomography (CT) scans.[9,11] A representative titanium cage is shown in **Fig. 2**.

Disclosure Statement: T.E. Mroz receives or has the right to receive royalty payments for invention(s) commercialized through Stryker Corporation. The other authors have nothing to disclose.
[a] Cleveland Clinic Lerner College of Medicine, Cleveland Clinic, 9500 Euclid Avenue, Cleveland, OH 44195, USA;
[b] Center for Spine Health, Cleveland Clinic, Desk S40, 9500 Euclid Avenue, Cleveland, OH 44195, USA
* Corresponding author.
E-mail address: mrozt@ccf.org

Neurosurg Clin N Am 31 (2020) 57–64
https://doi.org/10.1016/j.nec.2019.08.007
1042-3680/20/© 2019 Elsevier Inc. All rights reserved.

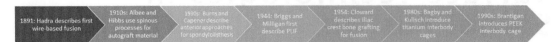

Fig. 1. Timeline of fusion interbody cage development.

A porous titanium alloy Ti-6Al-4V may have usefulness in addressing some of the limitations of pure titanium by decreasing its elastic modulus and facilitating bony ingrowth. Wu and colleagues[12] in a 2013 study used electron beam melting to develop a Ti-6Al-4V cage with 68.0% ± 5.3% porosity and an elastic modulus of 2.5 GPa. They implanted Ti-6Al-4V cages and PEEK control cages with bone autograft into the C3-C4 and C5-C6 disk spaces, respectively, of 1- to 2-year-old sheep. They found the porous Ti-6Al-4V cage had increased bone ingrowth at 3 months and 10 times the amount of bone apposition at 6 months after implantation compared with PEEK cages. The authors argue that the lower elastic modulus of this alloy is closer to that of native cortical bone and thus facilitated more natural load transfer, which can in turn stimulate bony ingrowth.[12] Furthermore, despite the porous nature of the Ti-6Al-4V cage, no fractures occurred in their study, indicating that the decrease in elastic modulus did not necessarily weaken the cage when applied under physiologic loading.

Wu and coauthors[12] found that surface enhancements to titanium such as roughness and porosity have been shown to enhance osseointegration through promoting increased levels of growth factors such as transforming growth factor-β1 and osteoprotegerin that contribute to bone formation. Indeed, Olivares-Navarrete and colleagues[13] in 2013 showed that rough titanium alloy discs showed increased osteogenic and angiogenic factors compared with smooth titanium alloy discs or PEEK discs. Textured Ti6Al4V implants also are associated with decreased expression of proinflammatory proteins such as IL-6, IL-8, and Toll-like receptor 4, as well as decreased expression of proteins associated with necrosis and apoptosis.[14] Olivares-Navarrete and colleagues[14] in their 2015 study suggest that the lack of integration seen with PEEK implants could be due to increased levels of these inflammatory and cellular damage-related factors.

Other authors have used different research methodologies to assess the role of porosity in surface technology. A study by Guyer and coauthors[15] in 2016 supports the usefulness of porosity in facilitating osseointegration with titanium. In their study, Guyer and colleagues[15] drilled 16 holes into each of 2 skulls of living swine and inserted porous titanium cylindrical pins, uncoated PEEK pins, or allograft pins. After 5 weeks, they humanely killed the animals and used an MTS machine (MTS Systems Corporation, Eden Prairie, MN) to measure the pull out strength of the pins.

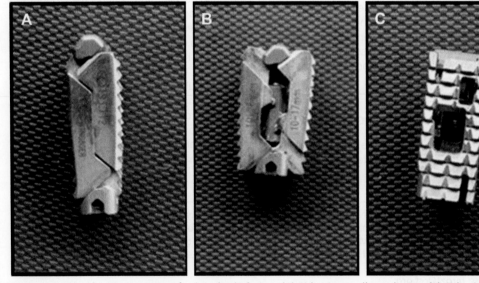

Fig. 2. Example of a titanium cage for interbody fusion. (*A*) Side view, collapsed cage. (*B*) Side view, expanded cage. (*C*) Front view.

They found the porous titanium scaffold pins had significantly higher pullout strength than the PEEK or allograft pins, likely owing to increased osseointegration facilitated by the porous meshwork.

Another technology that has been developed to facilitate interbody fusion is surface texturing. A 2012 study by Olivares-Navarrete and colleagues[16] compared smooth and microtextured Ti-6Al-4V and PEEK discs on their surface properties and ability to induce maturation of MG63 human osteoblast-like cells. They found that MG63 cells expressed more bone morphogenic proteins (BMP)2, BMP4, and BMP7 compared with PEEK, and that the surface roughness of Ti-6Al-4V induced more messenger RNA expression for BMP2 and BMP4, suggesting that roughness supports osteoblast maturation and may facilitate bone fusion.[16]

Although there is a paucity of high-level studies comparing the various titanium analogues, evidence for optimizing surface topography is drawn from animal models and basic science studies. Salou and colleagues[7] in 2015 showed that titanium implants coated with columnar TiO_2 nanotubes had higher pull out strengths at 4 weeks after implantation into the femoral condyles of New Zealand White Rabbits compared with microtextured titanium or PEEK. A study by Gittens and colleagues[6] in 2012 similarly found differentiation and maturation of primary human osteoblasts was increased when microscale and nanoscale roughness was present on TiAlV substrates. These small animal research models provide a good foundation in support of TiAlV technology; however, the clinical impact is not yet known.

POROUS TANTALUM

Tantalum has been used in clinical practice since the 1940s.[17] Although tantalum itself is bioinert, porous tantalum provides a scaffold for bony ingrowth, and the low elastic modulus similar to native trabecular bone may limit the effects of stress shielding and subsidence seen with titanium cages.[17] Tantalum has also been shown to facilitate osteoblast differentiation, and owing to its excellent biomechanical and biomaterial properties, tantalum may have clinical usefulness in spine fusion.[17,18] Papacci and colleagues[19] in 2016 presented a study where they retrospectively examined 99 patients undergoing 1- or 2-level anterior cervical discectomy and fusion (ACDF) who received porous tantalum cage implants. At the 5-year mark, they concluded that pain and quality of life scores significantly improved without major complications for 1- or 2-level fusion patients, suggesting that the safety of tantalum is not inferior when used for ACDF.[19]

Results obtained by Fernández-Fairen and co-authors[20] in 2019 reflect similar success in fusion rates with tantalum. In an 11-year follow-up study, the authors compared the outcomes of a porous tantalum cage and autologous bone grafting for ACDF on the factors of subsidence rates, adjacent segment degeneration, and segmental lordosis.[20] They found that the outcomes between tantalum and conventional autologous bone grafting were similar, with no statistically significant differences in the fusion rates. The authors state that the low Young's modulus relative to other implant materials such as titanium did not result in lower subsidence rates, but do conclude that long-term outcomes seen with tantalum cages are on par with those obtained with an iliac crest bone graft.

BIOACTIVE CERAMICS

Various technologies have been developed in the last 10 years to harness the strengths of older materials used in spine fusion while improving on their limitations, such as limited osseointegration in the case of PEEK or stress shielding and subsidence in the case of titanium. A representative PEEK cage is shown in **Fig. 3**.

Studies have been conducted in recent years with bioactive ceramics as disc spacers that feature both high strength and osseointegrative properties to facilitate bone fusion and decrease the need for a rigid cage. In 1 study, Lee and coauthors[21] fabricated spacers made of $CaO-SiO_2-P_2O_5-B_2O_3$, a material previously shown to be biocompatible and improve differentiation of mesenchymal stem cells, and implanted these spacers in patients requiring 1-level posterior lumbar interbody fusion for degenerative lumbar disk disease.[21,22] They randomized 86 patients undergoing 1-level posterior lumbar interbody fusion for lumbar spondylolisthesis to either the bioactive ceramic spacer or a titanium cage, and compared outcomes using the Oswestry Disability Index, Short Form-36, and visual analogue score scales at 3, 6, and 12 months after surgery. Seventy-five patients completed the study and follow-up, and although pain and disability decreased after surgery, no significant differences were observed in fusion between the groups at 12 months based on CT scanning. Therefore, although the $CaO-SiO_2-P_2O_5-B_2O_3$ spacer had similar fusion rates to the current standard titanium cage, the potentially increased cost of the bioactive ceramic may limit its therapeutic use in the near term.[22]

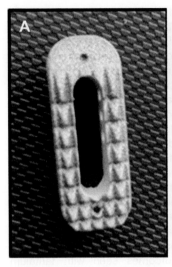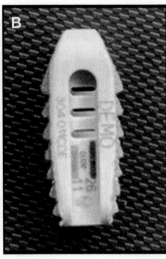

Fig. 3. PEEK cage for interbody fusion. (*A*) Front view. (*B*) Side view.

Pugely and coauthors[23] studied 45S5 bioactive glass as an adjunct to traditional iliac crest autograft to see whether the extender material facilitated arthrodesis in 69 mature New Zealand White rabbits. Because iliac crest bone grafting is associated with donor site morbidity, the authors compared traditional iliac crest bone grafting with a fibrillar collagen and tricalcium phosphate ceramic, and with 45S5 bioactive glass. The 3 groups had similar long-term fusion success at 12 weeks as measured by radiography, micro-CT scanning, and histologic assessment. However, the 45S5 group had an increased rate of fusion as seen at 4 weeks and 8 weeks, indicating that 45S5 glass may be therapeutically beneficial as an extender material to facilitate fusion and decrease donor site morbidity.[23]

Silicon nitride is another ceramic material thought to improve on some of the limitations of titanium and PEEK by offering osseoinductive capabilities without implant subsidence. Si_3N_4 has also been identified as a tough ceramic with favorable imaging characteristics.[24] Smith and coauthors[25] in 2018 retrospectively studied 58 patients who underwent ACDF and received a silicon nitride Si_3N_4 cage, and compared the outcomes of these patients with 34 who received fibular allograft spacers. They found that Si_3N_4 cages had a faster time to fusion and increased osseointegration over the allograft group. Further, Si_3N_4 cages had a lower subsidence than allograft spacers starting 3 months after surgery. The authors speculate that the increased fusion seen with Si_3N_4 is due to the release of silicic acid and ammonia that promote bone formation, as well as the presence of grain anisotropy that facilitates adhesion of eukaryotic cells.[25]

However, despite the favorable results seen in the study by Smith and colleagues,[25] the CASCADE trial comparing the results of a Si_3N_4 spacer with a PEEK cage for ACDF indicated no major clinical differences in outcome at 24 months after the operation. In the CASCADE trial, Arts and coauthors[24] enrolled 52 patients who received a Si_3N_4 spacer and 48 who received a PEEK cage. The authors did not observe a clinically significant difference in Neck Disability Index pain scores or fusion rates at 24 months, nor was a significant difference observed in subsidence.[24] The results obtained by Ball and coauthors[26] in a 2017 study reflect similar results. Ball and colleagues[26] retrospectively compared 20 patients receiving Si_3N_4 spacers for ACDF with patients receiving a traditional PEEK spacer. Although a modest decrease in flexion–extension angular rotation for the Si_3N_4 cohort was seen, this difference was not significant, and the authors reported both groups reaching 100% fusion at 3 years postoperatively.[26] Therefore, the additional advantage posed by Si_3N_4 cages remains controversial and a potential area of research interest.

HYBRID TECHNOLOGIES AND SURFACE COATING

There are advantages and disadvantages to both titanium and PEEK. Efforts have been made to harness the best of both of these materials and develop "hybrid" technologies. A variety of techniques have been developed to deposit titanium onto the surface of PEEK interbody cages to combine the radiolucency and favorable elastic modulus of PEEK with the osseointegrative potential of titanium. One such method is to use electron beam deposition, which is capable of creating a thin, uniform film of titanium at a low temperature on the surface of a PEEK implant.[27] In a 2010 study, Han and coauthors[27] used an e-beam evaporator to deposit titanium onto ultrasonically cleaned PEEK discs to a thickness of 1 μm. They then characterized the titanium surface including its crystalline structure and wettability, and found that there was twice the proliferation of osteoblasts in vitro on the Ti-coated PEEK discs compared with the untreated PEEK discs. Further, the Ti-coated PEEK disc had a significantly higher bone-in-contact ratio than the PEEK disc alone. These results demonstrate the potential benefits of titanium coating including maintenance of the underlying PEEK mechanical properties and enhanced osseointegrative potential compared with PEEK alone.[27]

Vacuum-plasma spraying is an alternative method to coat PEEK implants with titanium. High temperature spraying or chemical treatment of PEEK cages or carbon fiber PEEK cages would result in damage and exposure of the carbon fibers.[28] Thus, low-temperature vacuum spraying techniques have been developed to create rough titanium coatings between 6 and 12 microns.[28] In a 2018 study, Hoppe and coauthors[28] used a novel carbon-fiber PEEK cage in 42 patients undergoing 1- or 2-level TLIF and found that the Bridwell level I fusion rate at 24 months was 93.6%, with no patients experiencing radiolucency or pseudarthrosis. Although the study lacked a control group undergoing TLIF with alternate cage materials, the successful fusion of a Ti-coated carbon fiber PEEK cage was accomplished without the use of recombinant human BMP or iliac crest autologous bone grafting.

In a recent study, Makino and colleagues[29] evaluated the usefulness of Ti-coated PEEK in surgery for lumbar spine fusion. They used CT color mapping to evaluate bone ongrowth on Ti-coated PEEK cages in 24 patients who underwent 1- or 2-level posterior lumbar interbody fusion, and found that color CT mapping was adequate for studying bony ongrowth with good intraobserver and interobserver reliability. Bone ongrowth was seen in 134 of 248 surface images (54%) of interbody cages, and region of interest mapping was able to identify local increases in bone ongrowth as measured in Hounsfield units.

Cheng and coauthors[30] in 2018 evaluated biochemical markers such as BMP-2 and alkaline phosphatase transcription on plasma-sprayed Ti-PEEK compared with PEEK surfaces alone. They also compared in vivo biocompatibility by implanting 3 cylindrical rods of either sprayed or unsprayed PEEK in the hind legs of sheep and evaluated the pullout strength and bone apposition at 12 or 24 weeks after the operation.[30] The results showed that MG-63 osteoblast-like cells had increased adhesion and differentiation on Ti-PEEK substrates compared with PEEK alone, as well as upregulated levels of BMP-2 and alkaline phosphatase that indicate early bone formation. From the in vivo experiments, the pullout strength for Ti-PEEK implants was significantly higher than PEEK-only implants at both 12 and 24 weeks, indicating increased osseointegration and bone anchorage in the Ti-PEEK group.[30]

Titanium dioxide is also potentially beneficial as an alternative to pure titanium owing to the formation of OH^- groups that can bind Ca^{2+} and PO_4^{3-} ions to facilitate osseointegration.[31] In a 2015 study, Tsou and colleagues[31] investigated osseointegration of rutile and anatase titanium dioxide coatings applied via arc ion plating to PEEK implants in the femurs of male New Zealand white rabbits. They found that new lamellar bone had formed on the surface of the TiO_2/PEEK implants in 4 weeks, whereas the unmodified PEEK was covered with a fibrous layer of tissue. Further, as studied by pushout testing, the rutile TiO_2/PEEK implant had a shear strength of 6.51 MPa, more than double the shear strength of the unmodified PEEK implant.[31] The results of this study show that arc ion plated titanium dioxide may serve as a novel surface modification to increase osseointegration and mechanical fixation of spinal interbody implants.

Despite these benefits, Ti-coated PEEK cages can lead to a significant amount of wear debris accumulating around the implant, particularly when shear loading causes implant impaction.[32] In a 2016 study, Kienle and colleagues[32] obtained 6 Ti-coated PEEK interbody fusion cages and 6 made solely of surface-etched titanium. The cages were placed between polyurethane foam blocks mimicking vertebral bodies, and hit 2 to 4 times with a drop hammer to insert them. Wear particles were collected using plastic foil. The authors found that the Ti-coated PEEK implants gave off wear particles ranging from 1 to 191 μm in size, with most particles being less than 10 μm in diameter. Notably, only the coated implants gave off wear particles, and around one-half of the particles were at a size that they could be phagocytosed. This study raises a potential concern about the safety of Ti-coated PEEK implants because wear debris can lead to inflammatory reactions postoperatively.

SURFACE COATING WITH HYDROXYAPATITE

Hydroxyapatite (HA) is another material that may serve to increase the osseointegration of both

PEEK and titanium. In a 2005 study, Hasegawa and colleagues[33] evaluated pull-out forces of HA-coated titanium pedicle screws implanted into the L1 to L6 vertebrae of 2 female Beagle dogs. The 12 screws that received a HA coating had a significantly higher pull-out force than the titanium pedicle screws, and histologically were shown to have increased bone ingrowth, supporting the role of HA as a coating to increase bone fixation in interbody fusion devices.[33]

Results obtained by Johansson and colleagues[34] in 2016 showed PEEK coated with HA could also have similarly increased osseointegration. The authors implanted 1 PEEK screw coated with a 20- to 40-nm layer of HA and 1 pure PEEK screw into the femurs of 24 Swedish lop-eared rabbits and examined 12 of these rabbits at 3 weeks and 12 rabbits at 12 weeks postoperatively for histologic and morphologic changes in bone structure around the implants. They found that the HA-coated PEEK screws had higher bone-in-contact ratios at 3 and 12 weeks postoperatively than the native PEEK screws.[34] Thus, HA-coated PEEK may serve to increase integration of PEEK and reduce the complications of shear wearing and subsidence seen with titanium coatings and implants, respectively.

THREE-DIMENSIONAL PRINTING

In recent years, three-dimensional (3D) printing has seen a rapid increase in use in many different fields, including dentistry for maxillofacial implants,[35] aerospace for the manufacture of lightweight components,[36,37] and in medicine for the printing of orthopedic prostheses.[38] Given the versatility of the technology, recent efforts have focused on creating 3D-printed cages for spine fusion. A porous 3D titanium cage has the potential to address the limitation of Ti-coated PEEK cages giving off wear debris, while still allowing for osseointegration and decreasing range of motion. In their study, McGilvray and coauthors[9] evaluated bony ingrowth into a 3D-printed porous titanium cage in a sheep model. They performed spine fusion on L2 to L3 and L4 to L5 followed by placement of a PEEK, titanium-coated PEEK, or 3D-printed porous titanium alloy cage. After healing, sheep were humanely killed at 8 or 12 weeks after the operation, and spine specimens were analyzed using flexion–extension testing, micro-CT analysis, and histologic techniques. They found that PEEK implants were surrounded by dense fibrous connective tissue, demonstrating the PEEK-halo effect previously reported in the literature.[39] Further, the plasma-sprayed PEEK group showed less fibrous connective tissue and modest

Box 1
Surface modifications to base materials

Titanium
- Surface texturing
- Alloy Ti-6Al-4V
- Increased porosity via 3-dimensional printing

PEEK
- Ti coating
  - Vacuum-plasma spraying
  - TiO_2 coating via arc-ion plating
- Hydroxyapatite coating
- Ceramic or bioglass composite

neovascularization. The porous titanium alloy group demonstrated a statistically significant increase in stiffness, increased osteoblast activity, and increased bone–implant contact relative to the PEEK cages.[9] Wear-related complications were not observed in the porous titanium alloy group, which the authors believe is due to the lack of an interface between PEEK and titanium that have different elastic moduli.[9] Thus, porous titanium alloy cages may serve as an alternative to Ti-coated PEEK implants while limiting wear-related complications. **Box 1** lists some of the surface modifications discussed in this article.

SUMMARY

Questions remain as to the long-term outcomes in spine fusion as a function of interbody cage material or surface technology. Seaman and colleagues[40] in 2017 conducted a meta-analysis of 6 studies that compared titanium and PEEK cages for spine fusion. They found PEEK and titanium cages showed similar fusion rates, but titanium cages were associated with higher rates of subsidence. Importantly, none of the 6 studies included in the meta-analysis were Class I evidence, and the authors acknowledge that large randomized controlled trials are needed to verify whether a particular cage material is advantageous over the others.[40]

As mentioned by Seaman and coauthors,[40] few large-scale, randomized studies are available detailing the long-term outcomes of the various materials and surface modifications discussed in this review. PEEK seems to have lower subsidence rates than titanium, but titanium provides superior osseointegration. As for the newer technologies like porous titanium-coated PEEK, questions also remain about how best to apply this coating to native implants to decrease shear wearing and obtain optimal porosity. Other materials such as silicon nitride, tantalum, and bioactive glasses warrant further study as well.

Clinical outcomes studies in spine fusion seem to present conflicting results, partly owing to a paucity of randomized controlled trials comparing different cage materials and surgical techniques for fusion. Thus, more high-level data are needed that carefully consider patient demographics, surgical indications, and cage materials to clearly establish best practices in interbody fusion.

REFERENCES

1. Machado GC, Maher CG, Ferreira PH, et al. Trends, complications, and costs for hospital admission and surgery for lumbar spinal stenosis. Spine 2017; 42(22):1737–43.

2. Ghogawala Z, Dziura J, Butler WE, et al. Laminectomy plus fusion versus laminectomy alone for lumbar spondylolisthesis. N Engl J Med 2016;374(15): 1424–34.

3. Rao PJ, Pelletier MH, Walsh WR, et al. Spine interbody implants: material selection and modification, functionalization and bioactivation of surfaces to improve osseointegration: bioactivation of spine interbody implant surfaces. Orthop Surg 2014;6(2): 81–9.

4. Leong JC, Chow SP, Yau AC. Titanium-mesh block replacement of the intervertebral disk. Clin Orthop 1994;300:52–63.

5. Gittens RA, Olivares-Navarrete R, Cheng A, et al. The roles of titanium surface micro/nanotopography and wettability on the differential response of human osteoblast lineage cells. Acta Biomater 2013;9(4): 6268–77.

6. Gittens RA, Olivares-Navarrete R, McLachlan T, et al. Differential responses of osteoblast lineage cells to nanotopographically-modified, microroughened titanium–aluminum–vanadium alloy surfaces. Biomaterials 2012;33(35):8986–94.

7. Salou L, Hoornaert A, Louarn G, et al. Enhanced osseointegration of titanium implants with nanostructured surfaces: an experimental study in rabbits. Acta Biomater 2015;11:494–502.

8. Kurtz SM, Devine JN. PEEK biomaterials in trauma, orthopedic, and spinal implants. Biomaterials 2007; 28(32):4845–69.

9. McGilvray KC, Easley J, Seim HB, et al. Bony ingrowth potential of 3D-printed porous titanium alloy: a direct comparison of interbody cage materials in an in vivo ovine lumbar fusion model. Spine J 2018;18(7):1250–60.

10. Niu C-C, Liao J-C, Chen W-J, et al. Outcomes of interbody fusion cages used in 1 and 2-levels anterior cervical discectomy and fusion: titanium cages versus polyetheretherketone (PEEK) cages. J Spinal Disord Tech 2010;23(5):310–6.

11. McGilvray KC, Waldorff EI, Easley J, et al. Evaluation of a polyetheretherketone (PEEK) titanium composite interbody spacer in an ovine lumbar interbody fusion model: biomechanical, microcomputed tomographic, and histologic analyses. Spine J 2017; 17(12):1907–16.

12. Wu S-H, Li Y, Zhang Y-Q, et al. Porous titanium-6 aluminum-4 vanadium cage has better osseointegration and less micromotion than a poly-ether-ether-ketone cage in sheep vertebral fusion: porous Ti cage has better osseointegration than PEEK. Artif Organs 2013;37(12):E191–201.

13. Olivares-Navarrete R, Hyzy SL, Gittens RA, et al. Rough titanium alloys regulate osteoblast production of angiogenic factors. Spine J 2013;13(11):1563–70.

14. Olivares-Navarrete R, Hyzy SL, Slosar PJ, et al. Implant materials generate different peri-implant inflammatory factors: poly-ether-ether-ketone promotes fibrosis and microtextured titanium promotes osteogenic factors. Spine 2015;40(6):399–404.

15. Guyer RD, Abitbol J-J, Ohnmeiss DD, et al. Evaluating osseointegration into a deeply porous titanium scaffold: a biomechanical comparison with PEEK and allograft. Spine 2016;41(19):E1146–50.

16. Olivares-Navarrete R, Gittens RA, Schneider JM, et al. Osteoblasts exhibit a more differentiated phenotype and increased bone morphogenetic protein production on titanium alloy substrates than on poly-ether-ether-ketone. Spine J 2012;12(3):265–72.

17. Hanc M, Fokter SK, Vogrin M, et al. Porous tantalum in spinal surgery: an overview. Eur J Orthop Surg Traumatol 2016;26(1):1–7.

18. Sagomonyants KB, Hakim-Zargar M, Jhaveri A, et al. Porous tantalum stimulates the proliferation and osteogenesis of osteoblasts from elderly female patients. J Orthop Res 2011;29(4):609–16.

19. Papacci F, Rigante L, Fernandez E, et al. Anterior cervical discectomy and interbody fusion with porous tantalum implant. Results in a series with long-term follow-up. J Clin Neurosci 2016;33:159–62.

20. Fernández-Fairen M, Alvarado E, Torres A. Eleven-year follow-up of two cohorts of patients comparing stand-alone porous tantalum cage versus autologous bone graft and plating in anterior cervical fusions. World Neurosurg 2019;122:e156–67.

21. Lee JH, Seo J-H, Lee KM, et al. Fabrication and evaluation of osteoblastic differentiation of human mesenchymal stem cells on novel CaO-SiO$_2$-P$_2$O$_5$-B$_2$O$_3$ glass-ceramics: osteoblastic differentiation of hMSC. Artif Organs 2013;37(7):637–47.

22. Lee JH, Kong C-B, Yang JJ, et al. Comparison of fusion rate and clinical results between CaO-SiO2-P2O5-B2O3 bioactive glass ceramics spacer with titanium cages in posterior lumbar interbody fusion. Spine J 2016;16(11):1367–76.

23. Pugely AJ, Petersen EB, DeVries-Watson N, et al. Influence of 45s5 bioactive glass in a standard calcium phosphate collagen bone graft substitute on the posterolateral fusion of rabbit spine. Iowa Orthop J 2017;37:193–8.

24. Arts MP, Wolfs JFC, Corbin TP. Porous silicon nitride spacers versus PEEK cages for anterior cervical discectomy and fusion: clinical and radiological results of a single-blinded randomized controlled trial. Eur Spine J 2017;26(9):2372–9.

25. Smith MW, Romano DR, McEntire BJ, et al. A single center retrospective clinical evaluation of anterior cervical discectomy and fusion comparing allograft spacers to silicon nitride cages. J Spine Surg 2018;4(2):349–60.

26. Ball HT, McEntire B, Bal BS. Accelerated cervical fusion of silicon nitride versus PEEK spacers: a comparative clinical study. J Spine 2017;06(06).

27. Han C-M, Lee E-J, Kim H-E, et al. The electron beam deposition of titanium on polyetheretherketone (PEEK) and the resulting enhanced biological properties. Biomaterials 2010;31(13):3465–70.

28. Hoppe S, Albers C, Elfiky T, et al. First results of a new vacuum plasma sprayed (VPS) titanium-coated carbon/PEEK composite cage for lumbar interbody fusion. J Funct Biomater 2018;9(1):23.

29. Makino T, Kaito T, Sakai Y, et al. Computed tomography color mapping for evaluation of bone ongrowth on the surface of a titanium-coated polyetheretherketone cage in vivo: a pilot study. Medicine (Baltimore) 2018;97(37):e12379.

30. Cheng BC, Koduri S, Wing CA, et al. Porous titanium-coated polyetheretherketone implants exhibit an improved bone–implant interface: an in vitro and in vivo biochemical, biomechanical, and histological study. Med Devices (Auckl) 2018; 11:391–402.

31. Tsou H-K, Chi M-H, Hung Y-W, et al. In vivo osseointegration performance of titanium dioxide coating modified polyetheretherketone using arc ion plating for spinal implant application. Biomed Res Int 2015; 2015:1–9.

32. Kienle A, Graf N, Wilke H-J. Does impaction of titanium-coated interbody fusion cages into the disc space cause wear debris or delamination? Spine J 2016;16(2):235–42.

33. Hasegawa T, Inufusa A, Imai Y, et al. Hydroxyapatite-coating of pedicle screws improves resistance against pull-out force in the osteoporotic canine lumbar spine model: a pilot study. Spine J 2005;5(3):239–43.

34. Johansson P, Jimbo R, Naito Y, et al. Polyether ether ketone implants achieve increased bone fusion when coated with nano-sized hydroxyapatite: a histomorphometric study in rabbit bone. Int J Nanomedicine 2016;1435.

35. Dawood A, Marti BM, Sauret-Jackson V, et al. 3D printing in dentistry. Br Dent J 2015;219(11):521–9.

36. Joshi SC, Sheikh AA. 3D printing in aerospace and its long-term sustainability. Virtual Phys Prototyp 2015;10(4):175–85.

37. Petrick IJ, Simpson TW. 3D printing disrupts manufacturing: how economies of one create new rules of competition. Res-Technol Manag 2013;56(6): 12–6. https://doi.org/10.5437/08956308X5606193.

38. Eltorai AEM, Nguyen E, Daniels AH. Three-dimensional printing in orthopedic surgery. Iindeque BGP. Orthopedics 2015;38(11):684–7.

39. Phan K, Hogan JA, Assem Y, et al. PEEK-Halo effect in interbody fusion. J Clin Neurosci 2016;24: 138–40.

40. Seaman S, Kerezoudis P, Bydon M, et al. Titanium vs. polyetheretherketone (PEEK) interbody fusion: meta-analysis and review of the literature. J Clin Neurosci 2017;44:23–9.

Stem Cells and Spinal Fusion

Vivek P. Shah, BS[a],*, Wellington K. Hsu, MD[b]

KEYWORDS

- Spine fusion • Stem cell • Mesenchymal stem cells • Autologous • Allogeneic

KEY POINTS

- Spinal fusion surgery is performed when any neurologic or structural impairment takes place at the spinal column; however, current therapeutics result in nonunion and other complications.
- Current bone graft options include autograft, synthetics, demineralized bone matrix, and recombinant human bone morphogenetic protein, which all have their own limitations.
- The need for alternatives has led to explorations in bone marrow-derived mesenchymal stem cells because they have shown osteogenic properties facilitating bone growth and spinal fusion.
- Sources of bone mesenchymal stem cells are autologous and allogeneic.
- Clinical studies show that autologous and allogeneic bone mesenchymal stem cell sources result in high percentages of spinal fusion and is much less morbid than the current gold standard of autograft.

INTRODUCTION

Spinal fusions are performed when there is any neurologic or structural impairment to the spinal column that risks injury to the spinal cord.[1] Many pathologies exist that result in the need for stabilization including disc herniation, degenerative disk disease, tumor, spondylosis (which could result in radiculopathy and/or myelopathy), and trauma.[2,3] A successful spinal fusion surgery occurs when new bridging and stability of bone forms between the transverse processes of 2 or more adjacent vertebrae. What fuels this bone formation are osteogenic and biological agents that activate a series of cytokine and inflammation factors to induce bone formation.[4] Since 1990, lumbar spinal fusion procedures have increased by more than 220%, which is greater than that for knee and hip arthroplasty combined.[5]

There are a variety of spinal fusion procedures that are routinely performed depending on the anatomic location. The most common type, a posterolateral fusion, consists of bridging bone across the transverse processes and facet joints of these vertebrae.[6] Anterior approaches to the cervical and lumbar spine offer greater access to the disc and lead to a more complete discectomy when compared with a posterior equivalent. Lateral approaches have become more common recently, which affords disc space exposure through the retroperitoneal space via minimal access tubular technology. This type of procedure has the best indication for coronal deformity.

Nonunion occurs in spinal fusion cases at a rate of 25% to 30% depending on the procedure. Success depends on a number of variables, such as the patient's original bone volume and quality, surgical approach, and details of procedure.[7] Other factors include lower parent bone surface, tensile forces, and interference with surrounding musculature.[8] In patients where nonunion occurs, they often experience higher levels of pain, instability,

Disclosure Statement: The authors have nothing to disclose.
a Department of Orthopedic Surgery – Hsu Lab, Northwestern University, Chicago, IL 60611, USA;
b Northwestern Department of Orthopedic Surgery, 259 East Erie Street 13th Floor Lavin Family Pavilion, Chicago, IL 60611, USA
* Corresponding author. 408 Cromwell Place, Hopkinsville, KY 42240.
E-mail address: vshah1101@gmail.com

and an increase in cost and stress.[9] Patients at risk for pseudarthrosis include elderly, female, and a history of diabetes mellitus, thoracolumbar kyphosis, and/or metabolic bone disease.[10–13] Additionally, cigarette smoking is known to inhibit spinal fusion and cause higher rates of pseudarthrosis. Owing to such high variability, surgeons must decide on different treatment methods best suited for each patient and their history.

BONE GRAFT OPTIONS

The historic gold standard for bone graft has been the autologous harvest of bone, usually from the iliac crest or local bone from the surgical site. Autograft represents an ideal source because it is composed of osteogenic factors like collagen and bone minerals, osteoinductive factors like cytokines, and the family of beta transforming growth factors, as well as osteogenic components such as bone marrow stem cells or osteoblastic/preosteoblastic cells.[14] Despite autograft leading to a high successful fusion rate, there are morbidity and supply issues,[15] such as intraoperative blood loss and donor site morbidity.[16,17] Among the considerations is that the patient is also at risk for infections, hematomas, wound healing problems, possible fracture, and/or neurologic injuries.[18] Therapeutic solutions can obviate the need for autograft harvest, which can lead to better patient outcomes.

Currently, there are a number of bone graft substitute and extender categories that are available to surgeons. Some examples include synthetics, demineralized bone matrix (DBM), or growth factors such as recombinant human bone morphogenetic protein 2 (BMP)-2. All of these products have their own set of limitations and complications. For example, BMP can cause complications such as airway edema, severe inflammatory responses, radiculopathy, seroma and hematoma formation, osteolysis, and heterotopic bone formation.[19–21] DBM ensures the preservation of native bone proteins and growth factors in any new bone formation and is often used with other osteoconductive graft substitutes,[22,23] but it is unclear if it can fully support spinal fusion on its own.[24] Synthetic matrices such as hydroxyapatite have only been studied as a bone graft extender rather than a stand-alone substitute for bone graft.[25] There are still many more treatments to be evaluated.

The current landscape of spinal biologics has a clinical unmet need, which has led to ventures in stem cell therapy. Advances in regenerative medicine research has shown that bone marrow-derived mesenchymal stem cells (MSCs) have osteogenic properties that can result in spinal fusion. This property is mainly important because it is the less morbid option; the harvesting method is very simple and optimized to provide the 3 main components of osteogenesis.[26] However, the survival of the stem cells as well as biochemical control once implanted in to the body remains a huge challenge. Major advancements in the field of material sciences has created 3-dimensional structures that retain cells and provide nutrients for cell growth.[27] Further research will hopefully elucidate the exact mechanism of action of MSCs being osteogenic or osteoinductive.[15]

STEM CELL USE IN SPINAL FUSION

Stem cells, generally speaking, can be defined as "immature" tissue precursor cells that they can differentiate in to different types of cell lines that function at specific parts or systems of the body. The broad class of stem cells can be broken into 3 main groups: (i) embryonic stem cells from early age embryos, (II) induced pluripotent cells, and (iii) adult stem cells. Adult stem cells include MSCs, neural stem cells, and hematopoietic stem cells.[28]

Human mesenchymal cells from bone marrow were first discovered by Friedenstein and colleagues[29] in 1968 and described to be fibroblast-like, secreting cytokines and growth factors that contribute to hematopoiesis and many other processes. MSCs are often sourced from other adult tissues, including muscle[30] and subcutaneous fat.[31] These cells have also been shown to resist immunologic rejection and inhibit a range of immune cells including dendritic cells, macrophages, neutrophils, and T and B lymphocytes.[32,33] The greatest limitation for autologous stem cell use is derived from the method in which they are harvested. For example, bone marrow puncture does not allow for a plentiful supply of stem cells[34] and it has been shown that less than 1% of MSCs survive for more than 1 week after implantation.[35] Another drawback is that whenever there is more than 2 mL of bone marrow aspiration, this amount is usually diluted with peripheral blood, which decreases the overall concentration of MSCs.[36] Finally, this source of cells may be unreliable in the elderly population, explained by the effect of aging on dissipation of the potency of the stem cells.[37]

Adipose-derived MSCs can be autologous or allogeneic and extracted through liposuction, which is much less painful versus extracting from bone marrow aspiration.[38,39] Adipose-derived MSCs also demonstrate an increase of fusion levels, but much work remains to fully define this method before clinical applications can be used.[40] Embryonic stem cells have large capabilities to differentiate into many different cell lineages within all 3 germ layers; however, ethical concerns preclude its use in spine surgery.[27]

Allogeneic stem cells are those transplanted from a matching donor that are used to suppress some disease or restore some function to tissue. Allogeneic MSCs are usually harvested from some donor and stored and chemically altered in a laboratory for enhancement or characterization; however, some studies have shown concerns for immune reactions.[41] Allogeneic stem cell sources are important for cases where patients have low bone volume and will not be able to produce enough stem cells without possible complications, which may be common in the elderly population. Ultimately, allogeneic mesenchymal precursor cells have been used for disc regeneration and fusion enhancement.[42] Although this category of bone graft options has cornered a significant share of the market, there are few data available that demonstrate its definitive mechanism of action.

CLINICAL STUDIES

In a systematic review of clinical studies involving autologous and allogeneic stem cells, we identified 18 different clinical studies reporting the use of different types of stem cells mixed with different variants for spinal fusion (**Table 1**). Factors such as surgical approach, time point, fusion assessment, treatment conditions, stem cell type, and fusion rate were evaluated and used for inclusion in this review. These studies look at spinal fusion procedures such as posterolateral fusion, anterior cervical discectomy and fusion, posterior and anterior lumbar interbody fusion. Time points selected were either 12 months or 24 months and fusion assessment was either radiography or computed tomography scan.

All of the studies using autologous MSCs (n = 11) used bone marrow aspirate; however, each study involved a different carrier to support in bone growth stimulation. One of these trials included 41 patients undergoing posterolateral fusion for degenerative disc disease using enriched bone marrow aspirate with beta-tricalcium phosphate at a 24-month time point.[44] Ultimately, this resulted in a 95.1% fusion rate bilaterally evaluated using computed tomography. Another study using bone marrow concentrate with macroporous biphasic phosphate ceramics graft and autologous bone as the treatment source with 15 patients at a 24-month time point demonstrated 100% fusion visualized computed tomography scanning.[55] Another systematic review evaluated the results from 7 various clinical studies that compared autologous bone marrow aspirate with various carriers with either iliac crest or local bone graft. The carriers included collagen only, collagen and hydroxyapatite, hydroxyapatite and tricalcium phosphate, autograft, DBM, and biphasic calcium phosphates. The 2 groups that showed the highest fusion scores were the collagen only with bone marrow aspirate and the hydroxyapatite and tricalcium phosphate with bone marrow aspirate group with fusion rates of 100% and 98%, respectively. The collagen group was assessed for fusion using plain radiographs and the hydroxyapatite and tricalcium phosphate group used computed tomography.[56]

Studies involving allogeneic MSCs were fewer (n = 7). One study reported results in 52 patients undergoing either circumferential fusion, anterior lumbar interbody fusion, or transforaminal lumbar interbody fusion with Osteocel (Nuvasive, San Diego, CA), which is an allograft-based tissue containing live stem cells. Both radiographs and computed tomography scans were used for fusion evaluation, which was reported at 92.3%.[49] Osteocel has also been evaluated for spinal fusion using different carriers including DBM and autograft, which resulted in 89.6% and 85% fusion rates, respectively. Another study involving 40 patients undergoing anterior cervical discectomy and fusion used Trinity Evolution Viable Cellular Bone Matrix (Orthofix, Lewisville, TX) as an allogeneic stem cell source.[54] This product is a cellular bone allograft with matrix as well as demineralized cortical bone. Fusion rates using computed tomography were reported at 91.4%.[54] Both Osteocel and Trinity Evolution show high rates of fusion and could be potential spinal fusion allogeneic graft options.

Currently, there are 19 clinical trials involving spinal fusion and specifically stem cells listed on clinicaltrials.gov. Two are currently actively recruiting and one is enrollment through invitation. The 2 actively recruiting involve bone marrow aspirate stem cell concentrate and allograft versus BMP-2 and the other is a multicenter prospective study on degenerative spine disorders. Four have been terminated; however, one has produced results involving a human amniotic tissue-derived allograft. Once the data from these trials are fully published and analyzed, we can advance on our current knowledge of spinal fusion and enhance its clinical application. However, clinical studies must increase their emphasis on patient demographics and specific surgical approaches so that we fully understand the variability of stem cell interaction.

DISCUSSION

Efficacious spinal fusion therapeutics can potentially reduce morbidity while maintaining proper

Table 1
Clinical trials

Study, Year	No. of Patients	Surgical Approach	Time Point	Fusion Assessment	Conditions	Allogeneic vs Autologous	Fusion Percentage
Eastlack et al,[43] 2014	182	ACDF w/plating	24 mo	CT scan	Osteocel and PEEK interbody cage and anterior plating	Allogeneic	87
Gan et al,[44] 2008	41	PLF for DDD or TLF	24 mo	CT scan	Enriched BMA + BTCP	Autologous	95.10
Hostin et al, 2013	22	AIF	12 mo	CT scan	Col + BMA in carbon fiber cage	Autologous	87
Ammerman et al,[45] 2013	23	MITLIF	12 mo	Radiograph	Osteocel + DBM	Allogeneic	91.30
McAfee et al,[46] 2013	25	ELIF	24 mo	CT scan	Autograft/Osteocel	Allogeneic	85
Caputo et al,[47] 2013	30	ELIF	12 mo	CT scan	Osteocel + DBM	Allogeneic	89.60
Tohmeh et al,[48] 2012	40	ELIF	12 mo	Fluoroscopy-guided radiography and CT scan	Osteocel + DBM	Allogeneic	90.20
Kerr et al,[49] 2011	52	360 fusion, ALIF, TLIF	5–8 mo	Radiograph and CT scan	Osteocel	Allogeneic	92.30
Kitchel,[50] 2006	25	PLF, IF	24 mo	CT scan	Collagen + BMA (from ICBG)	Autologous	82
Neen et al, 2006	50	PLF/TLF/360 fusion	24 mo	Radiograph	Collagen/hydroxyapatite + BMA (from ICBG)	Autologous	91
Niu et al,[51] 2009	21	PLF	24 mo	CT scan	Autograft + BMA (from ICBG)	Autologous	88.5
Vaccaro et al, 2007	73	PLF	24 mo	Radiograph	DBM + BMA (from ICBG)	Autologous	65

Bansal et al,[52] 2009	30	PLF	12 mo	CT scan	Hydroxyapatite + TCP + BMA (from ICBG)	Autologous	98
Morro-Barrero et al, 2007	35	PLF	24 mo	Radiograph	Biphasic calcium phosphates + BMA (from local bone graft)	Autologous	84
Taghavi et al,[53] 2010	62	PLF	24 mo	Radiograph	Collagen + BMA (from local bone graft)	Autologous	100
Peppers et al,[54] 2017	40	ACDF	12 mo	CT scan	Trinity evolution viable cellular bone matrix	Allogeneic	91.4
Odri et al,[55] 2012	15	PLF	24 mo	CT scan	Bone marrow concentrate w/macroporous biphasic phosphate ceramics graft and autologous bone	Autologous	100
Hart et al	40	PLF	24 mo	CT scan	Bone marrow concentrate w/spongious allograft chips	Autologous	80

Abbreviations: ACDF, anterior cervical discectomy and fusion; ALIF, anterior lumbar interbody fusion; BMA, bone marrow aspirate; CT, computed tomography; ICBG, iliac crest bone graft; IF, interbody fusion; MITLIF, minimally invasive transforaminal lumbar interbody fusion; PLF, posterolateral fusion; TCP, tricalcium phosphate; TLF, thoracolumbar fascia; TLIF, transforaminal lumbar interbody fusion.

bone regenerative properties. MSCs have gained significant interest because of its availability, ease of use, and regenerative capabilities. Allogeneic stem cell use is an attractive option, especially for those patients with poor bone marrow quality, such as that of the elderly population. Although there are a plethora of preclinical data on the use of MSCs in spinal fusion, there needs to be more clinical studies to demonstrate efficacy in humans.

A critical component for the success of this bone graft category involves various scaffolds used with different types of stem cells and their effect on efficacy. There are some limitations to commercially available scaffolds, resulting in an inability to effectively regenerate new bone, including high costs, difficulty of handling, and ease of manufacturing. For example, type I bovine collagen is a commonly used biomaterial for these products. Other important characteristics for a scaffold include its biomechanical properties such as suitable space in the pores, or porosity. A recent study has shown that in polylactic-co-glycolic acid (PLGA) with a 90- to 250-μm pore size showed the optimal cell proliferation, compressive strength, and cell interconnectivity.[57] The manufacturing methods have also evolved in this space such as recent advancements in 3-dimensional printing technologies that can create new synthetic, osteogenic biomaterials.[58] One example of this has been dubbed hyperelastic bone, which is composed of 90% hydroxyapatite by weight and 10% PLGA, and has 50% material porosity with cell viability and proliferation. Preclinical data demonstrate rapid ossification and new bone growth without any additional biological factors, which may help to improve on the current limitations of scaffold use in spinal fusion.[59]

Future advances in research in carrier construction will exploit mechanical characteristics such as the strut angle and pore size. The way MSCs interact with different scaffold material must also be further analyzed, as well as the safety of bioengineered implanted cells containing osteoinductive factors. If research can fully optimize the scaffold with transplanted stem cells to improve spinal fusion and remove the need for autograft, then overall this surgery will become much less morbid, chances of pseudarthrosis will decrease, and results will improve drastically. As we await the completion of many preclinical and clinical trials on this subject, we are on the cusp of great discoveries in stem cells and spinal fusion.

SUMMARY

Autograft for spinal fusion has always been used as the gold standard and a control in most current-day research studies owing to its osteogenic, osteoconductive, and osteoinductive properties. The future of spinal fusion is heading toward usage proteins such as BMP-2 and/or MSCs and characterizing these in vitro to recreate spinal fusion and bone formation. Preclinical results with various growth factors like DBM and hydroxyapatite with BMP or MSCs have already shown equivalent if not higher fusion rates as autograft. Bone marrow aspirate also shows equivalent rates and is much less morbid than the autograft procedure, especially in elderly patients or younger patients with poor bone quality. Autologous or allogeneic MSCs can achieve union without side effects and overall have the potential to become the gold standard for bone graft augmentation.

REFERENCES

1. Robbins MA, Haudenschild DR, Wegner AM, et al. Stem cells in spinal fusion. Global Spine J 2017; 7(8):801–10.
2. Lee SB, Cho KS, Kim JY, et al. Hybrid surgery of multilevel cervical degenerative disc disease : review of literature and clinical results. J Korean Neurosurg Soc 2012;52(5):452–8.
3. Lopez MJ, McIntosh KR, Spencer ND, et al. Acceleration of spinal fusion using syngeneic and allogeneic adult adipose derived stem cells in a rat model. J Orthop Res 2009;27(3):366–73.
4. Boden SD. Overview of the biology of lumbar spine fusion and principles for selecting a bone graft substitute. Spine 2002;27(16 Suppl 1):S26–31.
5. Deyo RA, Gray DT, Kreuter W, et al. United States trends in lumbar fusion surgery for degenerative conditions. Spine 2005;30(12):1441–5 [discussion: 1446–7].
6. McAnany SJ, Baird EO, Qureshi SA, et al. Posterolateral fusion versus interbody fusion for degenerative spondylolisthesis: a systematic review and meta-analysis. Spine 2016;41(23):E1408–e1414.
7. Kim YJ, Bridwell KH, Lenke LG, et al. Pseudarthrosis in long adult spinal deformity instrumentation and fusion to the sacrum: prevalence and risk factor analysis of 144 cases. Spine 2006;31(20):2329–36.
8. Rao RD, Bagaria V, Gourab K, et al. Autograft containment in posterolateral spine fusion. Spine J 2008;8(4):563–9.
9. Dickson DD, Lenke LG, Bridwell KH, et al. Risk factors for and assessment of symptomatic pseudarthrosis after lumbar pedicle subtraction osteotomy in adult spinal deformity. Spine 2014;39(15):1190–5.
10. Hermann PC, Webler M, Bornemann R, et al. Influence of smoking on spinal fusion after spondylodesis surgery: a comparative clinical study. Technol Health Care 2016;24(5):737–44.

11. Buchlak QD, Yanamadala V, Leveque JC, et al. Complication avoidance with pre-operative screening: insights from the Seattle spine team. Curr Rev Musculoskelet Med 2016;9(3):316–26.

12. Kim YJ, Bridwell KH, Lenke LG, et al. Pseudarthrosis in primary fusions for adult idiopathic scoliosis: incidence, risk factors, and outcome analysis. Spine 2005;30(4):468–74.

13. Keaveny TM, Yeh OC. Architecture and trabecular bone - toward an improved understanding of the biomechanical effects of age, sex and osteoporosis. J Musculoskelet Neuronal Interact 2002;2(3):205–8.

14. Khan SN, Cammisa FP Jr, Sandhu HS, et al. The biology of bone grafting. J Am Acad Orthop Surg 2005;13(1):77–86.

15. Olabisi R. Cell-based therapies for spinal fusion. Adv Exp Med Biol 2012;760:148–73.

16. Hui CF, Chan CW, Yeung HY, et al. Low-intensity pulsed ultrasound enhances posterior spinal fusion implanted with mesenchymal stem cells-calcium phosphate composite without bone grafting. Spine 2011;36(13):1010–6.

17. Laurie SW, Kaban LB, Mulliken JB, et al. Donor-site morbidity after harvesting rib and iliac bone. Plast Reconstr Surg 1984;73(6):933–8.

18. Delecrin J, Takahashi S, Gouin F, et al. A synthetic porous ceramic as a bone graft substitute in the surgical management of scoliosis: a prospective, randomized study. Spine 2000;25(5):563–9.

19. Wong DA, Kumar A, Jatana S, et al. Neurologic impairment from ectopic bone in the lumbar canal: a potential complication of off-label PLIF/TLIF use of bone morphogenetic protein-2 (BMP-2). Spine J 2008;8(6):1011–8.

20. Robin BN, Chaput CD, Zeitouni S, et al. Cytokine-mediated inflammatory reaction following posterior cervical decompression and fusion associated with recombinant human bone morphogenetic protein-2: a case study. Spine 2010;35(23):E1350–4.

21. Tannoury CA, An HS. Complications with the use of bone morphogenetic protein 2 (BMP-2) in spine surgery. Spine J 2014;14(3):552–9.

22. Park JJ, Hershman SH, Kim YH. Updates in the use of bone grafts in the lumbar spine. Bull Hosp Jt Dis (2013) 2013;71(1):39–48.

23. Fu TS, Wang IC, Lu ML, et al. The fusion rate of demineralized bone matrix compared with autogenous iliac bone graft for long multi-segment posterolateral spinal fusion. BMC Musculoskelet Disord 2016;17:3.

24. Tilkeridis K, Touzopoulos P, Ververidis A, et al. Use of demineralized bone matrix in spinal fusion. World J Orthop 2014;5(1):30–7.

25. Spivak JM, Hasharoni A. Use of hydroxyapatite in spine surgery. Eur Spine J 2001;10(Suppl 2):S197–204.

26. Fu TS, Chang YH, Wong CB, et al. Mesenchymal stem cells expressing baculovirus-engineered BMP-2 and VEGF enhance posterolateral spine fusion in a rabbit model. Spine J 2015;15(9):2036–44.

27. Schroeder J, Kueper J, Leon K, et al. Stem cells for spine surgery. World J Stem Cells 2015;7(1):186–94.

28. Vizoso FJ, Eiro N, Cid S, et al. Mesenchymal stem cell secretome: toward cell-free therapeutic strategies in regenerative medicine. Int J Mol Sci 2017;18(9) [pii:E1852].

29. Friedenstein AJ, Chailakhjan RK, Lalykina KS. The development of fibroblast colonies in monolayer cultures of guinea-pig bone marrow and spleen cells. Cell Tissue Kinet 1970;3(4):393–403.

30. Zheng B, Cao B, Crisan M, et al. Prospective identification of myogenic endothelial cells in human skeletal muscle. Nat Biotechnol 2007;25(9):1025–34.

31. Crisan M, Yap S, Casteilla L, et al. A perivascular origin for mesenchymal stem cells in multiple human organs. Cell Stem Cell 2008;3(3):301–13.

32. Caplan AI. Why are MSCs therapeutic? New data: new insight. J Pathol 2009;217(2):318–24.

33. Lyons AB, Parish CR. Determination of lymphocyte division by flow cytometry. J Immunol Methods 1994;171(1):131–7.

34. Ohgushi H, Kitamura S, Kotobuki N, et al. Clinical application of marrow mesenchymal stem cells for hard tissue repair. Yonsei Med J 2004;45(Suppl):61–7.

35. Toma C, Wagner WR, Bowry S, et al. Fate of culture-expanded mesenchymal stem cells in the microvasculature: in vivo observations of cell kinetics. Circ Res 2009;104(3):398–402.

36. Muschler GF, Boehm C, Easley K. Aspiration to obtain osteoblast progenitor cells from human bone marrow: the influence of aspiration volume. J Bone Joint Surg Am 1997;79(11):1699–709.

37. Jing W, Smith AA, Liu B, et al. Reengineering autologous bone grafts with the stem cell activator WNT3A. Biomaterials 2015;47:29–40.

38. Risbud MV, Shapiro IM, Guttapalli A, et al. Osteogenic potential of adult human stem cells of the lumbar vertebral body and the iliac crest. Spine 2006;31(1):83–9.

39. Eltorai AE, Susai CJ, Daniels AH. Mesenchymal stromal cells in spinal fusion: current and future applications. J Orthop 2017;14(1):1–3.

40. Tang ZB, Cao JK, Wen N, et al. Posterolateral spinal fusion with nano-hydroxyapatite-collagen/PLA composite and autologous adipose-derived mesenchymal stem cells in a rabbit model. J Tissue Eng Regen Med 2012;6(4):325–36.

41. Crevensten G, Walsh AJ, Ananthakrishnan D, et al. Intervertebral disc cell therapy for regeneration: mesenchymal stem cell implantation in rat intervertebral discs. Ann Biomed Eng 2004;32(3):430–4.

42. Oehme D, Goldschlager T, Rosenfeld JV, et al. The role of stem cell therapies in degenerative lumbar

spine disease: a review. Neurosurg Rev 2015;38(3): 429–45.

43. Eastlack RK, Garfin SR, Brown CR, et al. Osteocel Plus cellular allograft in anterior cervical discectomy and fusion: evaluation of clinical and radiographic outcomes from a prospective multicenter study. Spine 2014;39(22):E1331–7.

44. Gan Y, Dai K, Zhang P, et al. The clinical use of enriched bone marrow stem cells combined with porous beta-tricalcium phosphate in posterior spinal fusion. Biomaterials 2008;29(29):3973–82.

45. Ammerman JM, Libricz J, Ammerman MD. The role of Osteocel Plus as a fusion substrate in minimally invasive instrumented transforaminal lumbar interbody fusion. Clin Neurol Neurosurg 2013;115(7): 991–4.

46. McAfee PC, Shucosky E, Chotikul L, et al. Multilevel extreme lateral interbody fusion (XLIF) and osteotomies for 3-dimensional severe deformity: 25 consecutive cases. Int J Spine Surg 2013;7:e8–19.

47. Caputo AM, Michael KW, Chapman TM, et al. Extreme lateral interbody fusion for the treatment of adult degenerative scoliosis. J Clin Neurosci 2013; 20(11):1558–63.

48. Tohmeh AG, Watson B, Tohmeh M, et al. Allograft cellular bone matrix in extreme lateral interbody fusion: preliminary radiographic and clinical outcomes. ScientificWorldJournal 2012;2012:263637.

49. Kerr EJ 3rd, Jawahar A, Wooten T, et al. The use of osteo-conductive stem-cells allograft in lumbar interbody fusion procedures: an alternative to recombinant human bone morphogenetic protein. J Surg Orthop Adv 2011;20(3):193–7.

50. Kitchel SH. A preliminary comparative study of radiographic results using mineralized collagen and bone marrow aspirate versus autologous bone in the same patients undergoing posterior lumbar interbody fusion with instrumented posterolateral lumbar fusion. Spine J 2006;6(4):405–11 [discussion: 411–2].

51. Niu CC, Tsai TT, Fu TS, et al. A comparison of posterolateral lumbar fusion comparing autograft, autogenous laminectomy bone with bone marrow aspirate, and calcium sulphate with bone marrow aspirate: a prospective randomized study. Spine 2009;34(25):2715–9.

52. Bansal S, Chauhan V, Sharma S, et al. Evaluation of hydroxyapatite and beta-tricalcium phosphate mixed with bone marrow aspirate as a bone graft substitute for posterolateral spinal fusion. Indian J Orthop 2009;43(3):234–9.

53. Taghavi CE, Lee KB, Keorochana G, et al. Bone morphogenetic protein-2 and bone marrow aspirate with allograft as alternatives to autograft in instrumented revision posterolateral lumbar spinal fusion: a minimum two-year follow-up study. Spine 2010; 35(11):1144–50.

54. Peppers TA, Bullard DE, Vanichkachorn JS, et al. Prospective clinical and radiographic evaluation of an allogeneic bone matrix containing stem cells (Trinity Evolution® Viable Cellular Bone Matrix) in patients undergoing two-level anterior cervical discectomy and fusion. J Orthop Surg Res 2017; 12(1):67.

55. Odri GA, Hami A, Pomero V, et al. Development of a per-operative procedure for concentrated bone marrow adjunction in postero-lateral lumbar fusion: radiological, biological and clinical assessment. Eur Spine J 2012;21(12):2665–72.

56. Hanna JH, Saha K, Jaenisch R. Pluripotency and cellular reprogramming: facts, hypotheses, unresolved issues. Cell 2010;143(4):508–25.

57. Kim HY, Kim HN, Lee SJ, et al. Effect of pore sizes of PLGA scaffolds on mechanical properties and cell behaviour for nucleus pulposus regeneration in vivo. J Tissue Eng Regen Med 2017;11(1):44–57.

58. Do AV, Khorsand B, Geary SM, et al. 3D printing of scaffolds for tissue regeneration applications. Adv Healthc Mater 2015;4(12):1742–62.

59. Jakus AE, Rutz AL, Jordan SW, et al. Hyperelastic "bone": a highly versatile, growth factor-free, osteoregenerative, scalable, and surgically friendly biomaterial. Sci Transl Med 2016;8(358):358ra127.

Cervical Disc Replacement

Jeremy Steinberger, MD[a], Sheeraz Qureshi, MD, MBA[b,*]

KEYWORDS

- Cervical disc replacement
- Arthroplasty
- Anterior cervical discectomy and fusion
- Cervical spine surgery

KEY POINTS

- Cervical disc replacement and anterior cervical discectomy and fusion are excellent techniques to treat cervical spine pathology.
- Cervical disc replacement preserves range of motion and avoid a fusion surgery.
- Owing to its preservation of segmental mobility, the potential to reduce the adjacent segment disease, and the lack of plating or harvesting bone graft, arthroplasty is as an excellent surgical option.
- The literature is growing in support of the success and longevity of arthroplasty and it is an important technique in a spine surgeon's armamentarium.

INTRODUCTION

Cervical spine surgery is a treatment option for patients with radiculopathy and/or myelopathy who suffer from cervical degenerative changes and have exhausted conservative measures. Anterior cervical discectomy and fusion (ACDF) has been the treatment of choice for anterior cervical surgery, but anterior cervical disc replacement (CDR), or arthroplasty, has been gaining significant momentum over the past 2 decades. ACDF is a fusion procedure, making it nonphysiologic, because it eliminates motion at the surgical level. In contrast, the ball-and-socket prosthesis design of arthroplasty has been shown to simulate normal motion in all 3 rotation planes at the level of surgery and replicates physiologic motion at the surgical site as well as the adjacent levels.[1] Range of motion after CDR is preserved and flexion–extension radiograph angles range from 5.7° to 10.6°.[2–5]

Although ACDF has been shown to be a safe and effective surgery over decades, CDR attempts to counter some of its negative aspects. ACDF carries a risk of pseudoarthrosis, at rates of 0% to 15.2%.[6] Additionally, patients can develop adjacent segment disease (ASD) after ACDF owing to altered biomechanical stresses on adjacent levels to surgery. A systematic review undertaken by Lawrence and colleagues[7] found ASD rates of 11% to 12% at 5 years, 16% to 38% at 10 years, and 33% at 17 years. Lee and colleagues[8] showed rates of adjacent segment reoperation after ACDF of 2.4% per year and showed that 22.2% of patients would need reoperation at adjacent segments by 10 years postoperatively. ACDF often involves plating, which can increase the risk of dysphagia owing to pressure on the esophagus and can lead to mechanical errors such as loosening of the plate or screws. Last, ACDF may involve the harvesting of iliac crest bone graft to increase fusion rates. Owing to its preservation of segmental mobility, the potential to decrease ASD, and the lack of plating or harvesting bone graft, arthroplasty is increasingly being viewed as an excellent surgical option. The literature is growing in support of the success and longevity of arthroplasty and it is

Disclosure Statement: Dr. Jeremy Steinberger: Has no disclosures. Dr. Sheeraz Qureshi: Currently receiving Consulting Fees from Stryker K2M, Globus Medical, Inc., Paradigm Spine; Royalties from RTI, Globus Medical Inc., Stryker K2M; Ownership Interest in Avaz Surgical, Vital 5; Medical/Scientific Advisory Board member at Spinal Simplicity, Lifelink.com; Board membership at Healthgrades, Minimally Invasive Spine Study Group; Honoraria from AMOpportunities. The other authors have nothing to disclose.

[a] Hospital for Special Surgery, 535 E. 70th Street, New York, NY 10021, USA; [b] Orthopaedic Surgery, Minimally Invasive Spinal Surgery, Hospital for Special Surgery, Weill Cornell Medical College, 1300 York Avenue, New York, NY 10065, USA
* Corresponding author.
E-mail address: sheerazqureshimd@gmail.com

Neurosurg Clin N Am 31 (2020) 73–79
https://doi.org/10.1016/j.nec.2019.08.009
1042-3680/20/© 2019 Elsevier Inc. All rights reserved.

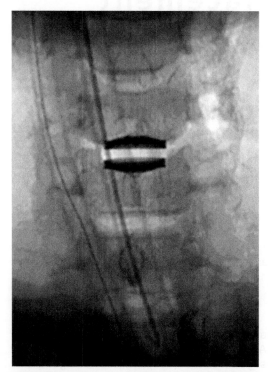

Fig. 1. Anteroposterior radiograph of a 1-level cervical disc replacement performed in a 39-year-old with myelopathic symptoms.

unquestionably an important technique in a spine surgeon's armamentarium.

INDICATIONS AND CONTRAINDICATIONS

Indications for CDR include 1- or 2-level cervical disc disease between C3 and C7 with a clinical

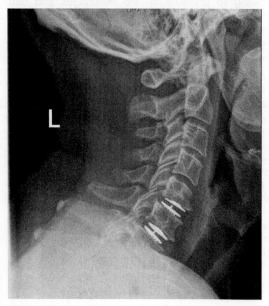

Fig. 2. Lateral radiograph of a 2-level CDR.

presentation of radiculopathy and/or myelopathy (**Figs. 1** and **2**).[9] Patients should not demonstrate instability (>3.5 mm translation on flexion–extension radiographs) because mobility preservation would not be desired.[10]

Contraindications to CDR include metabolic bone disease, active infection, known malignancy, allergy to the implant, and inflammatory spondyloarthropathy. Relative contraindications include kyphotic deformity, facet arthropathy, ankylosis, ossification of posterior longitudinal ligament, systemic disease, substantially collapsed disc space, and prior surgery at the level of surgery.[11]

SURGICAL TECHNIQUE AND PROCEDURE
Preoperative Planning

Before surgery, patients should undergo basic preoperative laboratory tests and medical clearance, if necessary. Cervical radiographs should be obtained to assess alignment, spondylosis, osteophytic change, and disc height.

Advanced imaging is recommended including flexion–extension radiographs, computed tomography scan, and MRI without contrast. Flexion–extension radiographs demonstrate instability. Computed tomography scans demonstrate bone quality, facet disease, osteophytic changes, disc calcification, and ossification of the posterior longitudinal ligament. MRI is the gold standard for revealing compression and stenosis of the neural elements, ligamentous hypertrophy, and inflammatory changes.

If the patient has had prior anterior cervical approaches or neck surgery, an ENT consult is recommended to workup the patient for asymptomatic unilateral recurrent laryngeal nerve paralysis. If there is preexisting vocal cord paralysis on 1 side, the surgeon should perform the same sided approach as the index surgery. Bilateral injuries to the recurrent laryngeal nerve could lead to requirement of a postoperative tracheostomy.

Preparation and Patient Positioning

General endotracheal anesthesia should be used for all cervical arthroplasty procedures. Care should be taken to avoid manipulation of the neck in cases of severe cord compression and awake fiberoptic intubation can be considered in these cases. The endotracheal tube should be taped to the opposite side of the surgical approach to prevent it from interfering with the draping.

Prophylactic antibiotics should be administered before making the incision. The patient should be positioned supine with the head in neutral position. Care should be taken to prevent the head from moving from this neutral position during the surgery. Our method of preference is tape across the forehead to secure the patient's head to the bed. Padding should be used at all bony prominences, particularly in thinner patients. Shoulders should be taped down to ensure radiographic visualization of the level of surgery, particularly in the lower subaxial cervical spine. Additionally, the end plates should be seen in parallel on fluoroscopy.

Surgical Approach

A standard anterior cervical approach should be used. The skin is incised and platysma sectioned. The superficial layer of the cervical fascia should be opened. Using blunt dissection, the avascular plane should be developed and widened between the sternocleidomastoid and carotid bundle laterally and the trachea and esophagus medial. Finger palpation can be used to confirm the disc space (hills of the discs and valleys of the anterior vertebrae bone) and radiographs should be taken to ensure correct level.

Surgical Procedure

The longus colli muscles are detached and retracted. A self-retaining retractor is placed. Vertebral body distraction pins are placed into the vertebral bodies above and below the disc. The annulus is incised and a complete discectomy performed. The uncovertebral joints should be identified bilaterally. The posterior longitudinal ligament should be resected until the ventral aspect of the spinal cord can be seen. Use of the drill should be minimized to prevent the creation of an environment in which fusion or heterotopic ossification (HO) can occur. The end plates should not be violated so as not to cause subsidence. Foraminal decompression should be ensured by feeling out the neural foramen with an instrument such as a nerve hook. Although the uncovertebral joints should be decompressed, the entire uncinate should not typically be resected because this maneuver can introduce motion and instability. Crucial to CDR is centering the arthroplasty and sizing appropriately. Meticulous attention to centering and sizing has been shown to be an important factor in the maintenance of segmental motion.[12]

Under fluoroscopic visualization, the appropriately sized CDR device should be selected and the implant should be tamped into place after trialing. Lateral and AP radiographs should be performed to confirm central placement of the arthroplasty. Once in place, all distraction pins (if used) should be removed. Before hemostasis and layered closure is performed, copious irrigation is recommended to rid the surgical site of all bone dust.

COMPLICATIONS AND MANAGEMENT
Complications Related to the Anterior Cervical Approach

The neck contains many vital structures and many of the potential morbidities involve the surrounding structures. As a general principle, using blunt techniques can prevent many of the complications that can arise in the anterior approach.

Vascular injuries of the initial steps of the surgery include damage to superficial veins (anterior or external jugular vein) or the deeper vessels; these include the carotid artery, internal jugular vein, or branches of the external carotid artery and vein. Injuries to the carotid artery or internal jugular are extremely rare but devastating and an urgent vascular surgery consult should be obtained in the event of an injury these structures.

Injury to the recurrent laryngeal nerve has been described as secondary to the anterior cervical approach. For this reason, some surgeons prefer a left-sided to a right-sided approach because the classic course of the recurrent laryngeal nerve course is more at risk with a right-sided approach, although injury to the nerve can happen on either side. Postoperative hoarseness can occur owing recurrent laryngeal nerve injury owing to retraction, swelling, or inadvertent sectioning during surgery.

Mild dysphagia is common after anterior cervical approaches owing to esophageal manipulation and retraction during the surgery (in addition to endotracheal tube placement). Typically, patients improve with a gradual increase in diet consistency as tolerated. Dysphagia at 2 years was shown to be less in CDR than ACDF, likely owing to decreased implant prominence and plating near the esophagus.[13] Esophageal perforation is exceedingly rare but dreaded approach related complication.

If milky and chylous fluid is seen in the field, this likely indicates injury to the thoracic duct, which typically runs lateral to the esophagus in the left sided prevertebral fascia. Although rare, this complication can be treated with intraoperative ENT consult, low-fat diet, and total parenteral nutrition.

Horner's syndrome (ptosis, miosis, and anhydrosis) can develop after anterior cervical approaches if there is damage to the sympathetic chain. The sympathetic chain lies along the longus colli lateral to the vertebral bodies and can be injured with the Bovie electrocautery if the exposure is taken too widely.

A postoperative neck hematoma can result in airway obstruction and compromise. In the worst case scenario, if there is a postoperative hematoma with significant external pressure on the airway, the anesthesia team may not be able to intubate the patient and gain airway access; in this rare setting, the hematoma must be emergently evacuated at bedside without delay. For this reason, meticulous hemostasis is recommended after CDR.

Complications of Cervical Disc Replacement

Vascular injuries at the level of the decompression and discectomy portion of the surgery include damage to the vertebral artery. This can occur during the foraminotomy portion of the surgery. Preoperative assessment of both vertebral arteries should be performed before surgery. If there is any question of a vertebral artery anomaly, duplication, deviation from the transverse foramen, a preoperative computed tomography angiogram should be performed. This complication is very rare but catastrophic as it can lead to significant blood loss and/or strokes. Emergent vascular surgery consult should be placed and a stent or vertebral sacrifice may be necessary. Direct repair is often very difficult in this location.

Venous bleeding can often be encountered during this portion of the surgery as well as veins can lie in the fat lateral to the spinal cord. This bleeding can often be stopped with a hemostatic agent and gentle compression. Neurologic injuries include damage to the spinal cord or nerve roots. Dural tears can occur during CDR surgery; these can be difficult to repair from the anterior approach.

Hardware complications for CDR include incomplete decompression, malposition (eg, kyphotic, off center), improper sizing, metallosis, subsidence, infection, and vertebral body fracture.[14]

Park and colleagues[15] analyzed 21 patients who underwent revision surgery for CDR. Of these, 17 were attributed to poor patient selection or indication-related, 7 to insufficient decompressions, 7 malpositions, 6 cases of subsidence, 3 osteolysis, and 1 postoperative infection.

POSTOPERATIVE CARE

Patients should receive less than 24 hours of antibiotics. Use of postoperative collar, obtaining standing radiographs before discharge, and use of postoperative steroids/nonsteroidal anti-inflammatory drugs are surgeon dependent.

OUTCOMES

In an AOSpine International survey assessing spine surgeon perspective of CDR use, 47.8% of spine surgeons used arthroplasty in their practice[16] and this number is likely increasing. More than 100,000 CDR procedures are performed in the United States annually.[17] The literature supporting CDR has been growing substantially. According

to a review of cervical arthroplasty, 23 randomized clinical trials and 8 regulatory investigational device exemption trials from the US Food and Drug Administration have been performed for CDR. Of the investigational device exemption trials, the vast majority were multicenter randomized controlled trials, surveying more than 20 sites.[18] The outcomes after CDR have been very optimistic.

Findlay and colleagues[19] performed a systematic review with meta-analysis of the data from 3160 patients across 14 randomized controlled trials and concluded that CDR is superior to ACDF in the short and medium term. CDR was shown to have improved scores in neck disability index, Short Form (SF)-36, dysphagia, and satisfaction. Gao and colleagues[20] compared CDR and ACDF for 2-level disease with 5 years of follow-up. In this series, there was no significant difference in Japanese Orthopaedic Association (JOA) score, visual analog score, or neck disability index. Range of motion was increased in the CDR group and ASD was decreased. MacDowall and colleagues[21] evaluated 3998 patients who underwent CDR versus ACDF for radiculopathy and discovered no clinically important difference in outcomes between the 2 procedures at 5 years of follow-up.

Adjacent Segment Disease

To date, the literature reports success in achieving the CDR's primary purpose to decrease rates of ASD that are seen in ACDF. In a meta-analysis investigating ASD after CDR versus ACDF, Xu and colleagues[22] concluded that CDR decreased the rate of ASD and reoperation. Zhu and colleagues[23] compared 14 randomized controlled trials with similar findings. In the aforementioned meta-analysis by Findlay and colleagues,[19] there was less ASD at both 2 years (short term) and between 4 and 7 years (medium to long term). In a meta-analysis of 20 prospective, randomized, controlled, multicenter studies, Latka and associates[24] found that CDR had lower rates of ASD at 60 months of follow-up. Skovrlj and colleagues[14] reviewed 1068 cervical arthroplasty levels operated with 2.3 years of follow-up and described a mean rate of reoperation of 1.0%, revision rate of 0.2%, and removal of CDR rate of 1.2%.

Heterotopic Ossification

HO, or bridging of bone between the end plates, can disturb the segmental motion that CDR is designed to uphold. Owing to the emphasis on motion preservation, the reporting of HO after arthroplasty has been investigated. HO rates vary across the literature, with some reporting high values of HO, such as 33.3% of CDR patients in the study undertaken by Gao and coworkers[20] and 37.7% (26 of 69 patients) in in the study undertaken by Li and associates.[25] In the larger randomized controlled trials that have been performed, lower rates of 10% to 12% have been described in 1- and 2-level CDR surgeries.[3,26,27]

Although these rates at first glance may seem alarming, the cause of HO as well its clinical relevance have not been fully elucidated; Li and colleagues[25] noted an increase in HO in spondylotic patients and concluded that HO likely represents an evolution of a degenerative process and not a complication of arthroplasty surgery. This group found that although HO did decrease range of motion, it did not impact clinical outcomes. Zhou and colleagues[28] similarly found no connection between HO after CDR with worsened neck disability index, neck pain, or arm pain.

Return to Work

Many studies have compared CDR and ACDF regarding return to work. Heller and colleagues[29] conducted a prospective, randomized, multicenter study and found that CDR patients returned to work 13 days earlier than fusion patients. Another study by Sundseth and colleagues[30] compared CDR and ACDF in a blinded and randomized multicenter trial, and patients in the arthroplasty group returned to work 2 weeks earlier than patients in the fusion group. A third prospective randomized controlled trial by Gornet and colleagues[31] found that CDR patients returned to work 40 days postoperatively, compared with 60 days in the patients who underwent fusion.

Quality of Life

An improvement in quality of life after cervical spine surgery is paramount and many studies have shown a demonstrable improvement in quality of life after both ACDF and CDR. Davis and colleagues[32] used the SF-12 scale in comparing health-related quality of life after ACDF versus arthroplasty for 2-level pathology. In their randomized controlled trial that spanned 24 sites, there was a statistically significant difference in SF-12 scores between arthroplasty and ACDF: at all postoperative collected time points, CDR patients had improved quality of life compared with the fusion group. Gornet and colleagues[33] conducted another RCT and concluded there was no statistically significant difference between the 2 in terms of quality of life as assessed by the SF-36.

Cost Effectiveness

Menzin and colleagues[34] used return to work and work productivity to compare cost effectiveness between CDR and ACDF. There were $431 saved with CDR compared with ACDF in direct costs; that is, $6987 per patient was saved in 2-year costs. Qureshi and colleagues[35] reported a saving of $4836 with CDRs in a 20-year cost projection analysis. Of note, this work assumed a 20-year longevity to the prosthesis. McAnany and associates[36] performed a cost-utility analysis and, again, found an improved cost effectiveness of arthroplasty over fusion with a total cost of $102,274 for CDR and $119,814 for fusion. Finally, Radcliff and colleagues[37] performed a retrospective review of prospectively collected data with a 4-year minimum follow-up and found that for patients with 1-level degenerative disc disease, factoring in the lower ASD and complication rates of CDR, CDR is a more cost effective and more efficient surgery than fusion.

SUMMARY

CDR is an excellent surgery for symptomatic cervical spine disease for the appropriately selected patient. Complication and readmission rates are low and multiyear outcomes studies have shown success with CDR.

REFERENCES

1. Puttlitz CM, Rousseau MA, Xu Z, et al. Intervertebral disc replacement maintains cervical spine kinetics. Spine 2004;29(24):2809–14.
2. Nabhan A, Steudel WI, Nabhan A, et al. Segmental kinematics and adjacent level degeneration following disc replacement versus fusion: RCT with three years of follow-up. J Long Term Eff Med Implants 2007;17(3):229–36.
3. Radcliff K, Davis RJ, Hisey MS, et al. Long-term evaluation of cervical disc arthroplasty with the Mobi-C© cervical disc: a randomized, prospective, multicenter clinical trial with seven-year follow-up. Int J Spine Surg 2017;11:31.
4. Phillips FM, Geisler FH, Gilder KM, et al. Long-term outcomes of the US FDA IDE prospective, randomized controlled clinical trial comparing PCM cervical disc arthroplasty with anterior cervical discectomy and fusion. Spine (Phila Pa 1976) 2015;40(10):674–83.
5. Coric D, Guyer RD, Nunley PD, et al. Prospective, randomized multicenter study of cervical arthroplasty versus anterior cervical discectomy and fusion: 5-year results with a metal-on-metal artificial disc. J Neurosurg Spine 2018;1-10.
6. Shriver MF, Lewis DJ, Kshettry VR, et al. Pseudoarthrosis rates in anterior cervical discectomy and fusion: a meta-analysis. Spine J 2015;15(9):2016–27.
7. Lawrence BD, Hilibrand AS, Brodt ED, et al. Predicting the risk of adjacent segment pathology in the

cervical spine: a systematic review. Spine (Phila Pa 1976) 2012;37:S52–64.

8. Lee JC, Lee SH, Peters C, et al. Adjacent segment pathology requiring reoperation after anterior cervical arthrodesis: the influence of smoking, sex, and number of operated levels. Spine (Phila Pa 1976) 2015;40(10):E571–7.

9. Mummaneni PV, Amin BY, Wu JC, et al. Cervical artificial disc replacement versus fusion in the cervical spine: a systematic review comparing long-term follow-up results from two FDA trials. Evid Based Spine Care J 2012;3(S 01):59–66.

10. Leven D, Meaike J, Radcliff K, et al. Cervical disc replacement surgery: indications, technique, and technical pearls. Curr Rev Musculoskelet Med 2017;10(2):160–9.

11. Chang CC, Huang WC, Wu JC, et al. The option of motion preservation in cervical spondylosis: cervical disc arthroplasty update. Neurospine 2018;15(4):296.

12. Tu TH, Wu JC, Huang WC, et al. The effects of carpentry on heterotopic ossification and mobility in cervical arthroplasty: determination by computed tomography with a minimum 2-year follow-up. J Neurosurg Spine 2012;16(6):601–9.

13. Skeppholm M, Olerud C. Comparison of dysphagia between cervical artificial disc replacement and fusion: data from a randomized controlled study with two years of follow-up. Spine 2013;38(24):E1507–10.

14. Skovrlj B, Lee DH, Caridi JM, et al. Reoperations following cervical disc replacement. Asian Spine J 2015;9(3):471.

15. Park JB, Chang H, Yeom JS, et al. Revision surgeries following artificial disc replacement of cervical spine. Acta Orthop Traumatol Turc 2016;50(6): 610–8.

16. Chin-See-Chong TC, Gadjradj PS, Boelen RJ, et al. Current practice of cervical disc arthroplasty: a survey among 383 AOSpine International members. Neurosurg Focus 2017;42(2):E8.

17. Nesterenko SO, Riley LH III, Skolasky RL. Anterior cervical discectomy and fusion versus cervical disc arthroplasty: current state and trends in treatment for cervical disc pathology. Spine 2012; 37(17):1470–4.

18. Health Quality Ontario. cervical artificial disc replacement versus fusion for cervical degenerative disc disease: a health technology assessment. Ont Health Technol Assess Ser 2019;19(3):1.

19. Findlay C, Ayis S, Demetriades AK. Total disc replacement versus anterior cervical discectomy and fusion: a systematic review with meta-analysis of data from a total of 3160 patients across 14 randomized controlled trials with both short-and medium-to long-term outcomes. Bone Joint J 2018; 100(8):991–1001.

20. Gao X, Yang Y, Liu H, et al. A comparison of cervical disc arthroplasty and anterior cervical discectomy and fusion in patients with two-level cervical degenerative disc disease: 5-year follow-up results. World Neurosurg 2019;122:e1083–9.

21. MacDowall A, Moreira NC, Marques C, et al. Artificial disc replacement versus fusion in patients with cervical degenerative disc disease and radiculopathy: a randomized controlled trial with 5-year outcomes. J Neurosurg Spine 2019;30(3):323–31.

22. Xu S, Liang Y, Zhu Z, et al. Adjacent segment degeneration or disease after cervical total disc replacement: a meta-analysis of randomized controlled trials. J Orthop Surg Res 2018;13(1):244.

23. Zhu Y, Zhang B, Liu H, et al. Cervical disc arthroplasty versus anterior cervical discectomy and fusion for incidence of symptomatic adjacent segment disease: a meta-analysis of prospective randomized controlled trials. Spine 2016;41(19): 1493–502.

24. Latka D, Kozlowska K, Miekisiak G, et al. Safety and efficacy of cervical disc arthroplasty in preventing the adjacent segment disease: a meta-analysis of mid-to long-term outcomes in prospective, randomized, controlled multicenter studies. Ther Clin Risk Manag 2019;15:531.

25. Li G, Wang Q, Liu H, et al. Postoperative heterotopic ossification after cervical disc replacement is likely a reflection of the degeneration process. World Neurosurg 2019;125. e1063–e8. [Epub ahead of print].

26. Lanman TH, Burkus JK, Dryer RG, et al. Long-term clinical and radiographic outcomes of the Prestige LP artificial cervical disc replacement at 2 levels: results from a prospective randomized controlled clinical trial. J Neurosurg Spine 2017;27(1):7–19.

27. Burkus JK, Traynelis VC, Haid RW, et al. Clinical and radiographic analysis of an artificial cervical disc: 7-year follow-up from the Prestige prospective randomized controlled clinical trial. J Neurosurg Spine 2014;21(4):516–28.

28. Zhou HH, Qu Y, Dong RP, et al. Does heterotopic ossification affect the outcomes of cervical total disc replacement? A meta-analysis. Spine 2015; 40(6):E332–40.

29. Heller JG, Sasso RC, Papadopoulos SM, et al. Comparison of BRYAN cervical disc arthroplasty with anterior cervical decompression and fusion: clinical and radiographic results of a randomized, controlled, clinical trial. Spine (Phila Pa 1976) 2009;34(2):101–7.

30. Sundseth J, Fredriksli OA, Kolstad F, et al. The Norwegian Cervical Arthroplasty Trial (NORCAT): 2-year clinical outcome after single-level cervical arthroplasty versus fusion–a prospective, single-blinded, randomized, controlled multicenter study. Eur Spine J 2017;26(4):1225–35.

31. Gornet MF, McConnell JR, Burkus JK, et al. Two-level cervical disc arthroplasty with prestige LP

disc versus ACDF: a prospective, randomized, controlled multicenter clinical trial with 24-month results. Spine J 2015;15(10 Supplement 1):130S.

32. Davis RJ, Kim KD, Hisey MS, et al. Cervical total disc replacement with the Mobi-C cervical artificial disc compared with anterior discectomy and fusion for treatment of 2-level symptomatic degenerative disc disease: a prospective, randomized, controlled multicenter clinical trial. Clinical article. J Neurosurg Spine 2013;19(5):532–45.

33. Gornet MF, Lanman TH, Burkus JK, et al. Cervical disc arthroplasty with the Prestige LP disc versus anterior cervical discectomy and fusion, at 2 levels: results of a prospective, multicenter randomized controlled clinical trial at 24 months. J Neurosurg Spine 2017;26(6):653–67.

34. Menzin J, Zhang B, Neumann PJ, et al. A health-economic assessment of cervical disc arthroplasty compared with allograft fusion. Tech Orthop 2010; 25(2):133–7.

35. Qureshi SA, McAnany S, Goz V, et al. Cost-effectiveness analysis: comparing single-level cervical disc replacement and single-level anterior cervical discectomy and fusion. J Neurosurg Spine 2013; 19(5):546–54.

36. McAnany SJ, Overley S, Baird EO, et al. The 5-year costeffectiveness of anterior cervical discectomy and fusion and cervical disc replacement: a Markov analysis. Spine (Phila Pa 1976) 2014;39(23):1924–33.

37. Radcliff K, Zigler J, Zigler J. Costs of cervical disc replacement versus anterior cervical discectomy and fusion for treatment of single-level cervical disc disease: an analysis of the Blue Health Intelligence database for acute and long-term costs and complications. Spine (phila Pa 1976) 2015;40(8): 521–9.

Enhanced Recovery in Spine Surgery and Perioperative Pain Management

Vikram Chakravarthy, MD[a], Hana Yokoi, BS[b], Mariel R. Manlapaz, MD[c],
Ajit A. Krishnaney, MD[a],*

KEYWORDS

- Enhanced recovery after surgery • Pain management • Spine surgery • Opioid
- Postoperative outcomes • Acetaminophen • Gabapentin • Analgesia

KEY POINTS

- Enhanced recovery after surgery is an interdisciplinary, multimodal approach to improve postoperative outcomes by applying multiple evidenced-based interventions.
- Multimodal analgesia begins preoperatively with the consumption of acetaminophen and gabapentin, and continues intraoperatively and postoperatively.
- Intraoperative medications include ketamine, ketorolac, epidural analgesia, bupivacaine liposome injectable suspension, and lidocaine.
- For patients undergoing spinal fusion, there was no difference in long term rates of spinal fusion found between groups provided with normal dose (<120 mg/d) nonsteroidal anti-inflammatory therapy versus those without nonsteroidal anti-inflammatory therapy.
- Enhanced recovery after surgery and chronic pain management in the surgical spine patient requires a multidisciplinary, team-based approach with increasing accountability from the patient.

INTRODUCTION

Enhanced recovery after surgery (ERAS) is an interdisciplinary, multimodal approach to improve postoperative outcomes by applying multiple evidenced-based interventions. These interventions are incorporated into preoperative, intraoperative, and postoperative protocols based on identified risk factors for high-risk patients and surgeries. These protocols have been shown to reduce complications, hospital stays by 30% to 50%, readmissions, and costs.[1–3] ERAS has been effective in other specialties such as colorectal and orthopedic surgery, showing decreased postoperative complications and outcomes.[1,3]

ERAS has been recently adapted for spine surgery at multiple institutions in the United States. The Hospital for Special Surgery showed decreased length of stay, reduced complications, and no readmissions in their cohort study looking at 15 standardized ERAS elements.[4] For lumbar spine fusions, there was decreased length of stay, decreased blood loss, and improved pain

Disclosure: The authors have nothing to disclose.
[a] Department of Neurosurgery, Cleveland Clinic, S40, Cleveland, OH 44195, USA; [b] Case Western Reserve University School of Medicine, S40, Cleveland, OH, USA; [c] Department of General Anesthesiology, Cleveland Clinic, E31, Cleveland, OH 44195, USA
* Corresponding author. Department of Neurosurgery, Cleveland Clinic, S40, 9500 Euclid Avenue, Cleveland, OH.
E-mail address: KRISHNA@CCF.ORG

Neurosurg Clin N Am 31 (2020) 81–91
https://doi.org/10.1016/j.nec.2019.08.010
1042-3680/20/© 2019 Elsevier Inc. All rights reserved.

control in a retrospective cohort performed by Wang and colleagues.[5] Other studies have identified decreased postoperative intensive care unit admissions, a shorter length of stay, reduced cost, and decreased opioid consumption throughout the duration of the hospital stay. In addition, some studies have shown improved mobilization and ambulation rates at the 1-month follow-up.[6–8] Ali and colleagues[7] identified additional postoperative benchmarks that were impacted positively by implementation of ERAS at University of Pennsylvania, including decreased urinary catheter use and decreased opioid consumption at the 1-month follow-up.

The recent opioid epidemic in the United states has seen drug overdoses triple from 1999 to 2014.[9] Sixty-three percent of drug overdose-related deaths in 2015 involved use of an opioid medication.[9] Narcotic-based postoperative protocols for pain management have contributed to the opioid epidemic with surgery being a key risk factor for chronic opioid use.[10,11] Despite focusing on this postoperative issue, studies continue to show that the management of postoperative pain requires significant modifications.[12,13] As a result, current practices in perioperative pain management must be addressed to reduce opioid use while improving pain control for patients. The Joint Commission recommends establishing protocols using "multi-modal adjuvant therapies," including nonopioid analgesics to decrease the dose of opioids needed for optimal pain control. The National Action Plan to Prevent Adverse Drug Events states that federal agencies should use evidence-based strategies to optimize safe opioid prescribing including "multimodal, team-based care" and non-opioid pharmacologic therapies to "personalize pain management." This multimodal approach is defined as 2 or more analgesic drugs that act via different mechanisms administered in conjunction[14] (Fig. 1). The American Society of Anesthesiologists Task Force recommends that multimodal pain management be used whenever possible.[14]

Improvements in pain management for spine surgery can play a significant role in decreasing opioid use and improving pain management. The potential impact of multimodal protocols to treat spine surgery pain is large, between 2001 to 2011 there was a 70% increase in the overall number of spine surgeries.[10] A 2018 study showed that patients undergoing minimally invasive spine surgery consumed less than one-half the opioids they were prescribed postoperatively.[15] These results highlight the need for continuous monitoring and evaluation of patient pain management needs to decrease unnecessary opioid prescriptions. This finding has positive implications for

decreasing a patient's risk of opioid dependence, as well as decreasing the possibility of opioid diversion.[15] Implementation of protocols and reducing the quantity of opioids necessary for adequate pain control will only further reduce the quantity of opioids prescribed after hospital discharge.

Decreased opioid use is not only beneficial in decreasing drug-related adverse outcomes such as addiction, diversion, or death, but also advantageous for outcomes in spine surgery. Animal models have shown decreased rates of healing and fusion with opioid use.[16] In spine surgery, higher opioid prescriptions are associated with an increased risk of deep venous thrombosis, postoperative infection, gastrointestinal and respiratory complications, increased hospital length of stay, and higher overall hospital costs.

The ERAS paradigm is an ideal framework in which to incorporate the needed changes in postoperative pain management for spine surgery. Using evidence-based and best practice principles, rational pain management protocols can and have been created. ERAS pain management protocols emphasize a multidisciplinary approach across the operative episode to improve pain control and minimize narcotic consumption. One such protocol has been developed at the Cleveland Clinic and can serve as an example of an evidence-based rational spine surgery pain management protocol.

PREOPERATIVE PAIN MANAGEMENT INTERVENTIONS

Preemptive analgesia has been shown to reduce postoperative pain and narcotic consumption (Fig. 2). ERAS pain protocols therefore, should include preemptive analgesia on the day of surgery before initiation of the operation. A number of medications have been shown to be helpful preoperatively, including acetaminophen, gabapentin, and cyclooxygenase (COX)-2 inhibitors.

Acetaminophen

Multiple studies have demonstrated benefit of acetaminophen as part of a greater multimodal pain management protocol. The American Society of Anesthesiologists recommend administering scheduled acetaminophen with a maximum dose not to exceed 4 g/d to prevent the risk of hepatotoxicity.[14]

The benefits of acetaminophen include decreased opioid use, increased analgesic control, and more cost-effective care.[17] After lower extremity surgery, the addition of preoperative acetaminophen has been shown to decrease

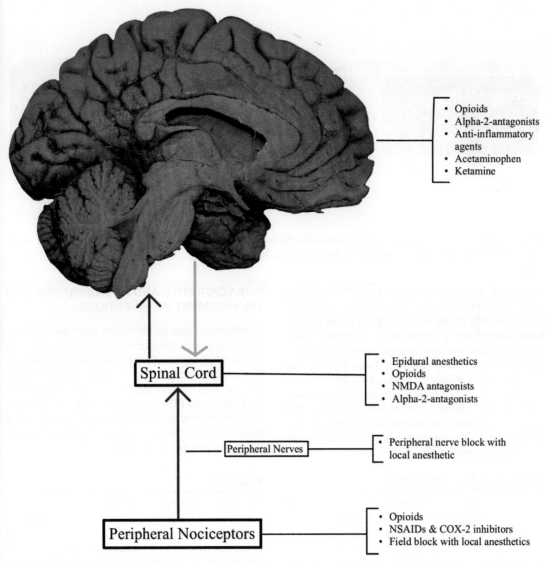

- Opioids
- Alpha-2-antagonists
- Anti-inflammatory agents
- Acetaminophen
- Ketamine

Spinal Cord
- Epidural anesthetics
- Opioids
- NMDA antagonists
- Alpha-2-antagonists

Peripheral Nerves
- Peripheral nerve block with local anesthetic

Peripheral Nociceptors
- Opioids
- NSAIDs & COX-2 inhibitors
- Field block with local anesthetics

Fig. 1. A representation of various levels of analgesia from the site of local tissue manipulation to the feedback loop in the central nervous system.

opioid consumption and reduce the need for analgesic rescue.[18] This low-cost analgesic medication provides effective pain relief after surgery, indicating a cheaper alternative.[19] A systematic review of acetaminophen in combination with nonsteroidal anti-inflammatory drugs (NSAIDS) by Ong and colleagues[20] demonstrates superior analgesia compared with either drug alone. Acetaminophen has few contraindications including severe liver disease, and few drug interactions. Current recommendations advise administering oral acetaminophen over intravenous (IV) administration with some studies showing little benefit of IV infusion.[17,21] However, there is controversy in the literature, with studies indicating a clear benefit

that has been corroborated by a Cochrane review of 75 studies presenting high-quality evidence.[22–24]

Gabapentin

Gabapentin has been shown to decrease pain scores, decrease morphine use, and decrease rates of postoperative nausea, vomiting, and pruritis with minimal side effects.[25–28] The significant decrease in postoperative nausea and vomiting provides additional justification for its use as a preemptive measure.[29] Other studies have confirmed decreased rates of opioid consumption without additional side effects and decreased rates of

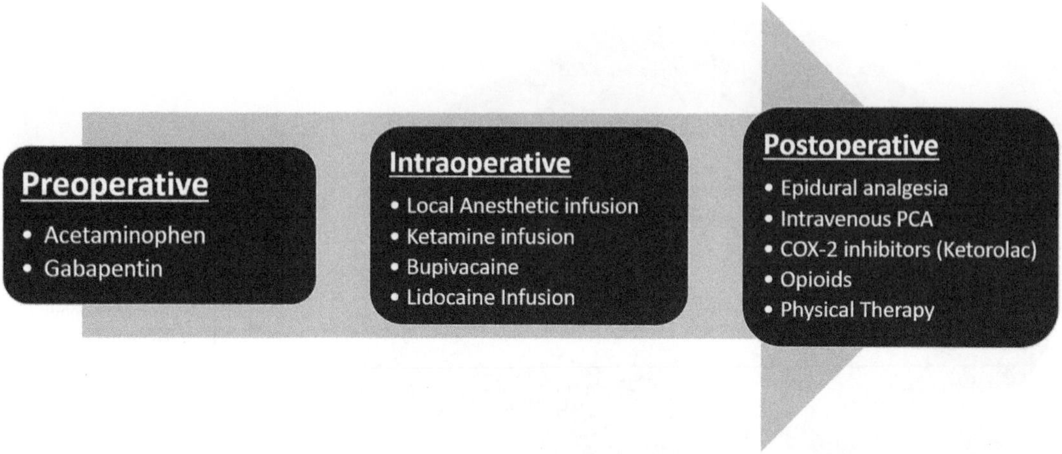

Preoperative
- Acetaminophen
- Gabapentin

Intraoperative
- Local Anesthetic infusion
- Ketamine infusion
- Bupivacaine
- Lidocaine Infusion

Postoperative
- Epidural analgesia
- Intravenous PCA
- COX-2 inhibitors (Ketorolac)
- Opioids
- Physical Therapy

Fig. 2. Schematic representation of the progression from preoperative to intraoperative to postoperative medications available for administration. PCA, patient-controlled analgesia.

the use of rescue pain medications.[30,31] Hegarty and Shorten[31] in a randomized placebo-controlled trial found that a single dose of pregabalin decreased postoperative morphine consumption, with an absolute difference of 42.3%. Gabapentin not only prevents hyperalgesia, but also acts as an anxiolytic, addressing the association between preoperative anxiety and postsurgical pain.[25] Based on these findings, The American Society of Anesthesiologists recommends that gabapentin be administered in the perioperative period.[14]

Cyclooxygenase-2 Inhibitors

The use of COX-2 inhibitors has had a significant impact on postoperative pain control when administered before surgery.[32] This is mediated by a decrease in prostaglandin synthesis, decreased tissue inflammation, and by preventing the sensitization of nociceptive receptors.[25] Furthermore, these agents are preferred to nonselective COX inhibitors owing to the preservation of platelet function and decreased risk of gastric bleeding. COX-2 inhibitors were not shown to increase the risk of bleeding in the perioperative period and have a decreased incidence of gastrointestinal side effects compared with nonselective NSAIDs.[33]

The American Society of Anesthesiologists Task Force recommends COX-2 inhibitors and nonselective NSAIDS to be added to the perioperative pain management regimen.[14] Pain management protocols combining COX-2 inhibitors and gabapentin have been shown to have effective analgesic control, improved patient satisfaction, and decreased opioid use with fewer side effects when compared with gabapentin monotherapy as found by Vasigh and colleagues.[34]

INTRAOPERATIVE AND POSTOPERATIVE PAIN MANAGEMENT INTERVENTIONS

An effective intraoperative pain management protocol requires collaboration with anesthesiology to create a rational multimodal series of intraoperative interventions to improve postoperative pain control. This collaboration is an integral aspect of the multimodal ERAS protocol. Various intraoperative specifications were delineated to aid in the postoperative management of all patients undergoing elective spine surgery.

Ketamine

The American Society of Anesthesiologists Task Force recommends the use of ketamine combined with IV morphine, which has demonstrated improved pain scores, decreased analgesic use, and improved nausea scores compared with IV morphine alone.[14] Previous studies have shown ketamine infusions to be effective in spine surgery and other surgical specialties with improved pain control and decreased opioid use.[35,36] A systematic review by Laskowski and colleagues[36] found ketamine to be of particular benefit in painful procedures, including upper abdominal, thoracic, and major orthopedic procedures. Pendi and colleagues[35] reviewed a total of 14 randomized controlled trials, finding supplemental perioperative ketamine to decrease postoperative opioid consumption up to 24 hours postoperatively in spine surgical patients.

The use of ketamine is recommended for patients with chronic pain owing to its opioid-sparing effect. Therefore, this therapy confers the greatest advantage in the patient population that is expected to require high doses of postoperative opioids.[36] Major side effects include neuropsychiatric symptoms and postoperative nausea and vomiting.

Lidocaine

Intraoperative IV lidocaine infusion has been shown to improve pain outcomes, decrease hospital length of stay, and has been associated with a decreased 30-day complication rate.[37,38] The clinical effects of lidocaine, by attenuation of the proinflammatory system to decrease pain and ileus, may outlast the infusion by hours or days.[39] This pain attenuation has an opioid-sparing effect and additionally reduces postoperative nausea and vomiting. These effects have been demonstrated in multilevel and major spine surgery where infusions resulted in decreased postoperative pain, decreased opioid consumption, and improved functional outcomes.[39]

Ketorolac

Ketorolac is an IV NSAID that has demonstrated significant effectiveness in controlling postoperative pain and decreasing opioid consumption when administered perioperatively. It is typically given at the end of the case and continued into the postoperative period. For patients younger than 65 years of age, a 30-mg dose is given; patients 65 and older a 15-mg bolus is given. Contraindications for administration include a creatinine of more than 1.3 mg/dL, a bleeding disorder, or surgeon discretion based on intraoperative hemostasis.

The American Society of Anesthesiologists Task Force recommends NSAIDs to be administered around the clock, with improved pain scores when IV morphine is combined with ketorolac compared with IV morphine alone.[14] A meta-analysis by Gobble and colleagues[40] demonstrated that ketorolac was equivalent to opioids for pain control after surgery and should be administered in the perioperative period to decrease opioid use. In a randomized, double-blind trial by Cepeda and colleagues,[41] adding 30 mg IV of ketorolac to an analgesic regimen for treating postoperative pain decreased morphine rescue dose requirements and opioid-related side effects in the early postoperative period.

Ketorolac and spinal fusion

For patients undergoing spinal fusion, there was no difference in long-term rates of spinal fusion found between groups provided with normal dose (<120 mg/d) NSAID therapy versus those without NSAID therapy.[32] A meta-analysis showed that normal dose NSAID exposure for less than 2 weeks after spinal fusion does not have adverse effects on fusion rates; however, high doses (>120 mg/d) of ketorolac were associated with impaired spinal fusion rates.[42] In animal models, NSAIDs have also been shown to significantly inhibit fracture healing process; however, these effects depend on their timing, dose, and duration, supporting the recommendation that they should only be administered for short periods.[43]

Ketorolac and hemostasis

Interestingly, the only side effect that has been documented to occur with single-dose or short-term administration of ketorolac is increased operative site bleeding after surgical procedures with raw surface areas (eg, tonsillectomy, adenoidectomy, total joint replacements, and major plastic surgery).[44] There are no controlled studies in the peer-reviewed literature demonstrating an increase in blood loss during or after surgery when standard doses of ketorolac were administered at the end of surgery or in the early postoperative period. It is our practice for the anesthesiologist to confirm with the surgeon before ketorolac administration and withhold the dose if there were any intraoperative concerns with hemostasis.

Ketorolac and renal failure

The transient decrease in renal function postoperative is clinically insignificant for patients with normal renal function. There is no greater risk of acute renal failure when administered for short periods in the acute postoperative setting. However, patients with preexisting low creatinine clearance may be at greater risk for postoperative renal failure.[45]

Narcotic Analgesia

Short-acting narcotic anesthetic agents such as remifentanil, fentanyl, or sufentanil are routinely given intraoperatively during surgery to provide intraoperative analgesia. Remifentanil has consistently been shown to induce hyperalgesia in the 24 hours after surgery.[46] However, based on a randomized controlled trial by de Hoogd and colleagues[47] in the cardiac surgery literature, it is suggested that intraoperative administration is associated with increased narcotic use for up to 3 months postoperatively. Using long-acting IV narcotics intraoperatively can provide analgesia that extends into the immediate postoperative period, thereby diminishing the need for rescue narcotic doses in the recovery room.

Epidural Analgesia

In a meta-analysis by Wu and colleagues,[48] epidural analgesia provided a statistically and clinically significant improvement in postoperative pain control compared with IV patient-controlled analgesia with opioids regardless of analgesic regimen, measured pain outcomes, type of epidural analgesia, or surgical site. Attempts at enhancing the analgesic potential of patient-controlled analgesia demonstrated that a combination solution (local anesthetic with opioid) compared with opioid alone resulted in improved pain scores but greater motor weakness. Patients who received infusions of opioid alone had greater amount of pruritus.[14] Epidural analgesia (combination solution) provides more significant analgesia and higher patient satisfaction compared with IV patient-controlled analgesia after spinal fusion surgery.[49] In addition, it has been found to decrease postoperative opioid consumption. Contraindications include occurrence of intraoperative durotomy and/or if the epidural space is deemed too small to advance an epidural catheter (eg, multiple revisions or fibrosis of epidural space). Analgesic infusion begins in the postanesthetic care unit once a stable neurologic examination has been obtained.

Local Anesthetics

The American Society of Anesthesiologists Task Force recommends regional blockade with local anesthetic.[14] Meta-analysis of randomized controlled trials report improved pain scores and decreased analgesic use with preincisional infiltration of ropivacaine and bupivacaine.[49]

Recently, liposomal bupivacaine (Exparel), an amide local anesthetic that targets the voltage gated sodium ion channels, has emerged as an extended release form that may last up to 72 hours after infiltration. Since its approval by the US Food and Drug Administration, it has been used in thoracic, orthopedic, and abdominal surgeries, demonstrating decreased pain, decreased opioid requirement, and improved patient satisfaction.[49] In spine surgery liposomal bupivacaine was shown to decrease pain in the immediate postoperative period and decrease the total opioid consumption.[5,49] The formulation used in the United States encapsulates the drug in liposomes made of biodegradable cholesterols that breakdown slowly over a desired time period.[50,51] It is our practice to infiltrate the incision before skin closure with a combination of both liposomal bupivacaine and marcaine to provide both immediate and delayed pain relief.

Nonpharmacologic Interventions for Pain Management

Nonpharmacologic interventions that have been used to manage postoperative pain include preoperative counseling with cognitive–behavioral therapy, biofeedback visualization, and chiropractic manipulation (**Fig. 3**). A case series by Archer and colleagues[51] reviewed 8 postoperative patients who suffered from a high fear of movement who underwent 6-session cognitive-behavioral–based physical therapy. This therapy addresses the fear of movement through behavior self-control and cognitive restructuring techniques aiming to increase physical activity. At the 6-month follow-up, 7 patients demonstrated a clinically significant decrease in pain and all 8 patients had significant reduction in disability. This was quantified by 5 patients demonstrating clinically significant improvement on the 10-m walk test. Nicholls and colleagues[52] found 6 papers in their systematic review citing a decrease in postoperative pain disability and intensity in cognitive–behavioral therapy–based psychological interventions.

Biofeedback therapy encourages relaxation and helps to alleviate various conditions associated with stress. In a case series of Taiwanese patients after total knee arthroplasty, Wang and colleagues[53] found that the group receiving biofeedback training twice daily for 5 days demonstrated significantly less pain from continuous passive motion therapy compared with the control group. Although pain is a subjective measure, this modality may offer patients an additional option when seeking nonpharmacologic care.

In a European study of patients undergoing surgical correction of adolescent idiopathic scoliosis,

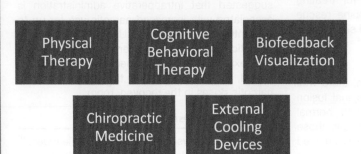

Fig. 3. The nonpharmacologic interventions available to patients during the postoperative period to decrease the use of narcotic medications.

a novel cooling brace was used postoperatively to minimize opioid consumption. The Game Ready device is connected to an external circuit with ice cold water cooled to 4°C. The brace is applied in the postanesthetic care unit and is kept on for 24 hours. Bellon and colleagues[54] found that in their consecutive cohort of 22 patients, the cooling brace allowed for decreased opioid use after surgical correction in children.

Early Mobilization

All patients are mobilized by nursing staff within 8 hours of arriving to the regular nursing floor. If the patient is unable to mobilize an automatic physical therapy order is sent out. High-risk patients receive a physical therapy evaluation automatically to ensure maximal mobilization and recovery. It is encouraged to remove the urinary catheter early in the postoperative period (ie, postoperative day 1). Prolonged immobilization has deleterious effects on pulmonary function and decreases the integrity of muscles, the urinary tract, and the skin. Immobilization prolongs hospital stay and carries an increased risk of deep venous thrombosis, pulmonary embolism, pulmonary infection, and urinary tract infections. Early mobilization has been shown to decrease perioperative complications and decrease length of stay by 34%. Additionally, patients mobilized early were more likely to be discharged to home.

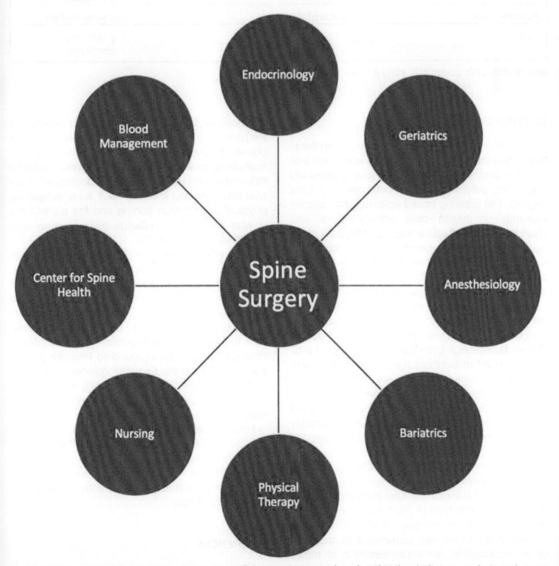

Fig. 4. A schematic of the various components of the ERAS protocol at the Cleveland Clinic Foundation, demonstrating the multidisciplinary approach.

Table 1
Pain-specific ERAS protocol at the Cleveland Clinic

Morning of Surgery		Acetaminophen			Gabapentin
Dose		1 g PO			300–600 mg PO

	Ketamine	Lidocaine IV	Ketorolac	Epidural Analgesia	Local Anesthetic at incision Site
Pre-incision	0.25 mg/kg bolus	1.5 mg/kg bolus			Lidocaine 1% 1 mL/kg or 2.5 mg/kg max dose
During surgery	5 µg/kg/min infusion	1.5 mg/kg/h infusion			
After closure			15–30 mg IV bolus	Fentanyl morphine	0.25% bupivacaine 1 mL/kg or 2.5 mg/kg max

Postoperative		Ketorolac			Acetaminophen
Dose		<120 mg/d for 72 h			1 g q6h until discharge

Abbreviations: PO, per os; q6h, every 6 hours.

DISCUSSION

Enhanced recovery after spine surgery is an iterative, innovative systems-based care approach that has demonstrated effectiveness and statistically significant outcomes at different tiers of care (**Fig. 4**). The growing opioid epidemic has placed pressure on health care administrators and providers to find effective non-narcotic, pain management options for postoperative patients. Multimodal analgesia has been shown in the literature across different health care disciplines to decrease opioid consumption and improve postoperative mobilization. As discussed, there are various pharmacologic and nonpharmacologic perioperative interventions available to patients (**Table 1**). Although previous studies have identified the need to overhaul the postoperative pain management regimen of patients undergoing surgery, few data have been published on the most effective strategy to do so. Various ERAS protocols have been published citing standardization as a common theme leading to improved outcomes.

Although the creation of a standardized, iterative protocol is possible, there are challenges to implementation and compliance. One such challenge to implementing this type of program is compliance owing to individual surgeon preference and a limited ability to monitor adherence to the program. Additionally, the implementation of multilevel reforms makes for difficult analysis for causation with the potential for a variety of confounding factors. The various components of the protocol may need to be introduced in different phases to improve compliance. Working across multiple disciplines is a potential barrier owing to different methods of charting and decreased inter-specialty communication. Pain is a subjective physical examination finding and the subjectivity is what drives the challenge to both study and effectively treat the entity.

The effectiveness of ERAS protocols at improving outcomes, efficiency, and patient satisfaction remains to be seen. Early studies of ERAS protocols have shown that implementation of a multitiered approach to improving patient outcomes is possible, and may be effective and beneficial to the surgical spine patient. Multidisciplinary collaboration has been found to improve patient and provider satisfaction with greater confidence that each aspect of the patient's preoperative and postoperative care benchmarks has been met.

Future studies are needed to analyze efficiency, efficacy, and cost effectiveness. Emerging research and innovation will help to determine the optimal protocols to use the various pain management options available to the clinician today.

REFERENCES

1. Wainwright Thomas W, Immins T, Middleton Robert G. Enhanced recovery after surgery

(ERAS) and its applicability for major spine surgery. Best Pract Res Clin Anaesthesiol 2016;30(1): 91–102.

2. Ljungqvist O, Scott M, Fearon Kenneth C. Enhanced recovery after surgery. JAMA Surg 2017;152(3):292.

3. Gustafsson Ulf O, Hausel J, Thorell A, et al. Adherence to the enhanced recovery after surgery protocol and outcomes after colorectal cancer surgery. Arch Surg 2011;146(5):571–7.

4. Soffin EM, Vaishnav AS, Wetmore D, et al. Design and implementation of an enhanced recovery after surgery (ERAS) program for minimally invasive lumbar decompression spine surgery: initial experience. Spine (Phila Pa 1976) 2019;44(9): E561–70.

5. Wang MY, Chang P-Y, Grossman J. Development of an Enhanced Recovery After Surgery (ERAS) approach for lumbar spinal fusion. J Neurosurg Spine 2017;26(4):411–8.

6. Grasu Roxana M, Cata Juan P, Dang Anh Q, et al. Implementation of an Enhanced Recovery After Spine Surgery program at a large cancer center: a preliminary analysis. J Neurosurg Spine 2018; 29(5):588–98.

7. Ali ZS, Flanders TM, Ozturk AK, et al. Enhanced recovery after elective spinal and peripheral nerve surgery: pilot study from a single institution. J Neurosurg Spine 2019;1–9. https://doi.org/10. 3171/2018.9.SPINE18681.

8. Dagal A, Bellabarba C, Bransford R, et al. Enhanced perioperative care for major spine surgery. Spine (Phila Pa 1976) 2018;1. https://doi.org/10.1097/ BRS.0000000000002968.

9. Rudd Rose A, Seth P, David F, et al. Increases in drug and opioid-involved overdose deaths - United States, 2010-2015. MMWR Morb Mortal Wkly Rep 2016;65(50–51):1445–52.

10. Dunn Lauren K, Yerra S, Fang S, et al. Incidence and risk factors for chronic postoperative opioid use after major spine surgery: a cross-sectional study with longitudinal outcome. Anesth Analg 2018;127(1): 247–54.

11. Kelly MA. Current postoperative pain management protocols contribute to the opioid epidemic in the United States. Am J Orthop (Belle Mead NJ) 2015; 44(10 Suppl):S5–8.

12. Apfelbaum Jeffrey L, Chen C, Mehta Shilpa S, et al. Postoperative pain experience: results from a national survey suggest postoperative pain continues to be undermanaged. Anesth Analg 2003;97(2): 534–40. table of contents.

13. Gan Tong J, Habib Ashraf S, Miller Timothy E, et al. Incidence, patient satisfaction, and perceptions of post-surgical pain: results from a US national survey. Curr Med Res Opin 2014;30(1):149–60.

14. American Society of Anesthesiologists Task Force on Acute Pain Management. Practice guidelines for acute pain management in the perioperative setting: an updated report by the American Society of Anesthesiologists Task Force on Acute Pain Management. Anesthesiology 2012;116(2): 248–73.

15. Tan WH, Yu J, Feaman S, et al. Opioid medication use in the surgical patient: an assessment of prescribing patterns and use. J Am Coll Surg 2018; 227(2):203–11.

16. Jain N, Himed K, Toth JM, et al. Opioids delay healing of spinal fusion: a rabbit posterolateral lumbar fusion model. Spine J 2018;18(9): 1659–68.

17. Schwenk Eric S, Mariano Edward R. Designing the ideal perioperative pain management plan starts with multimodal analgesia. Korean J Anesthesiol 2018;71(5):345–52.

18. Khalili G, Janghorbani M, Saryazdi H, et al. Effect of preemptive and preventive acetaminophen on postoperative pain score: a randomized, double-blind trial of patients undergoing lower extremity surgery. J Clin Anesth 2013;25(3):188–92.

19. Toms L, McQuay Henry J, Derry S, et al. Single dose oral paracetamol (acetaminophen) for postoperative pain in adults. Cochrane Database Syst Rev 2008;(4):CD004602.

20. Ong CK, Seymour RA, Lirk P, et al. Combining paracetamol (acetaminophen) with nonsteroidal antiinflammatory drugs: a qualitative systematic review of analgesic efficacy for acute postoperative pain. Anesth Analg 2010;110(4):1170–9.

21. Hiller A, Helenius I, Nurmi E, et al. Acetaminophen improves analgesia but does not reduce opioid requirement after major spine surgery in children and adolescents. Spine (Phila Pa 1976) 2012; 37(20):E1225–31.

22. McNicol ED, Ferguson MC, Haroutounian S, et al. Single dose intravenous paracetamol or intravenous propacetamol for postoperative pain. Cochrane Database Syst Rev 2016;(5):CD007126.

23. Mitra S, Carlyle D, Kodumudi G, et al. New advances in acute postoperative pain management. Curr Pain Headache Rep 2018;22(5):35.

24. Jebaraj B, Maitra S, Baidya DK, et al. Intravenous paracetamol reduces postoperative opioid consumption after orthopedic surgery: a systematic review of clinical trials. Pain Res Treat 2013;2013: 402510.

25. Nir R-R, Nahman-Averbuch H, Moont R, et al. Preoperative preemptive drug administration for acute postoperative pain: a systematic review and meta-analysis. Eur J Pain 2016;20(7):1025–43.

26. Arumugam S, Lau CS, Chamberlain RS. Use of preoperative gabapentin significantly reduces

postoperative opioid consumption: a meta-analysis. J Pain Res 2016;9:631–40.

27. Peng C, Li C, Qu J, et al. Gabapentin can decrease acute pain and morphine consumption in spinal surgery patients: a meta-analysis of randomized controlled trials. Medicine (Baltimore) 2017;96(15): e6463.

28. Liu B, Liu R, Wang L. A meta-analysis of the preoperative use of gabapentinoids for the treatment of acute postoperative pain following spinal surgery. Medicine (Baltimore) 2017;96(37):e8031.

29. Grant MC, Betz M, Hulse M, et al. The effect of preoperative pregabalin on postoperative nausea and vomiting: a meta-analysis. Anesth Analg 2016; 123(5):1100–7.

30. Kim JC, Choi YS, Kim KN, et al. Effective dose of peri-operative oral pregabalin as an adjunct to multimodal analgesic regimen in lumbar spinal fusion surgery. Spine (Phila Pa 1976) 2011;36(6):428–33.

31. Hegarty DA, Shorten GD. A randomised, placebo-controlled trial of the effects of preoperative pregabalin on pain intensity and opioid consumption following lumbar discectomy. Korean J Pain 2011; 24(1):22.

32. Siribumrungwong K, Cheewakidakarn J, Tangtrakulwanich B, et al. Comparing parecoxib and ketorolac as preemptive analgesia in patients undergoing posterior lumbar spinal fusion: a prospective randomized double-blinded placebo-controlled trial. BMC Musculoskelet Disord 2015; 16(1):59.

33. Sinatra R. Role of COX-2 inhibitors in the evolution of acute pain management. J Pain Symptom Manage 2002;24(1 Suppl):S18–27.

34. Vasigh A, Jaafarpour M, Khajavikhan J, et al. The effect of gabapentin plus celecoxib on pain and associated complications after laminectomy. J Clin Diagn Res 2016;10(3):UC04–8.

35. Pendi A, Field R, Farhan S-D, et al. Perioperative ketamine for analgesia in spine surgery: a meta-analysis of randomized controlled trials. Spine (Phila Pa 1976) 2018;43(5):E299–307.

36. Laskowski K, Stirling A, McKay WP, et al. A systematic review of intravenous ketamine for postoperative analgesia. Can J Anaesth 2011; 58(10):911–23.

37. Kim K-T, Cho D-C, Sung J-K, et al. Intraoperative systemic infusion of lidocaine reduces postoperative pain after lumbar surgery: a double-blinded, randomized, placebo-controlled clinical trial. Spine J 2014;14(8):1559–66.

38. Farag E, Ghobrial M, Sessler DI, et al. Effect of perioperative intravenous lidocaine administration on pain, opioid consumption, and quality of life after complex spine surgery. Anesthesiology 2013; 119(4):932–40.

39. Dunn Lauren K, Durieux Marcel E. Perioperative use of intravenous lidocaine. Anesthesiology 2017; 126(4):729–37.

40. Gobble RM, Hoang HL, Kachniarz B, et al. Ketorolac does not increase perioperative bleeding: a meta-analysis of randomized controlled trials. Plast Reconstr Surg 2014;133(3):741–55.

41. Cepeda MS, Carr DB, Miranda N, et al. Comparison of morphine, ketorolac, and their combination for postoperative pain: results from a large, randomized, double-blind trial. Anesthesiology 2005; 103(6):1225–32.

42. Li Q, Zhang Z, Cai Z. High-dose ketorolac affects adult spinal fusion: a meta-analysis of the effect of perioperative nonsteroidal anti-inflammatory drugs on spinal fusion. Spine (Phila Pa 1976) 2011;36(7): E461–8.

43. Geusens P, Emans Pieter J, de Jong Joost JA, et al. NSAIDs and fracture healing. Curr Opin Rheumatol 2013;25(4):524–31.

44. Marret E, Flahault A, Samama C-M, et al. Effects of postoperative, nonsteroidal, antiinflammatory drugs on bleeding risk after tonsillectomy: meta-analysis of randomized, controlled trials. Anesthesiology 2003;98(6):1497–502.

45. Lee A, Cooper MG, Craig JC, et al. Effects of nonsteroidal anti-inflammatory drugs on postoperative renal function in adults with normal renal function. Cochrane Database Syst Rev 2007;(2): CD002765.

46. Santonocito C, Noto A, Crimi C, et al. Remifentanil-induced postoperative hyperalgesia: current perspectives on mechanisms and therapeutic strategies. Local Reg Anesth 2018;11:15–23.

47. de Hoogd S, Ahlers Sabine JGM, van Dongen Eric PA, et al. Randomized Controlled Trial on the Influence of Intraoperative Remifentanil versus Fentanyl on Acute and Chronic Pain after Cardiac Surgery. Pain Pract 2018;18(4):443–51.

48. Wu CL, Cohen Seth R, Richman Jeffrey M, et al. Efficacy of postoperative patient-controlled and continuous infusion epidural analgesia versus intravenous patient-controlled analgesia with opioids: a meta-analysis. Anesthesiology 2005;103(5): 1079–88 [quiz: 1109-10].

49. Schenk Michael R, Putzier M, Kügler B, et al. Postoperative analgesia after major spine surgery: patient-controlled epidural analgesia versus patient-controlled intravenous analgesia. Anesth Analg 2006;103(5):1311–7.

50. Malik O, Kaye Alan D, Kaye A, et al. Emerging roles of liposomal bupivacaine in anesthesia practice. J Anaesthesiol Clin Pharmacol 2017;33(2): 151–6.

51. Archer KR, Motzny N, Abraham CM, et al. Cognitive-behavioral-based physical therapy to improve

surgical spine outcomes: a case series. Phys Ther 2013;93(8):1130–9.

52. Nicholls JL, Azam MA, Burns LC, et al. Psychological treatments for the management of postsurgical pain: a systematic review of randomized controlled trials. Patient Relat Outcome Meas 2018;9:49–64.

53. Wang T-J, Chang C-F, Lou M-F, et al. Biofeedback relaxation for pain associated with continuous passive motion in Taiwanese patients after total knee arthroplasty. Res Nurs Health 2015;38(1): 39–50.

54. Bellon M, Michelet D, Carrara N, et al. Efficacy of the Game Ready® cooling device on postoperative analgesia after scoliosis surgery in children. Eur Spine J 2019. https://doi.org/10.1007/s00586-019-05886-6.

Imaging Technologies in Spine Surgery

Vikram Chakravarthy, MD, Shehryar Sheikh, BA, Eric Schmidt, MD, Michael Steinmetz, MD*

KEYWORDS

- Spine imaging • Exoscope • Augmented reality • Visualization • Spine navigation • Microscope
- Virtual reality • Endoscope

KEY POINTS

- Many endoscope systems allow for the use of visualization modes that permit real-time digital enhancement of the image based on preset optimized modes of illumination, contrast enhancement, and color shifting.
- Although it may not completely replace the operative microscope's proven utility and reliability at this point in time, the cost, ergonomics, and uniform visualization benefits of the exoscope are attractive, especially at teaching hospitals.
- Augmented reality (AR), defined as adding digital elements to a live view by using a camera, is an emerging imaging technology in spine surgery.
- Spine surgeons are using virtual reality (VR)–based stimulators to become facile in the technical nuances of various procedures, including pedicle screw placement, vertebroplasty, and facet joint injection.
- Mixed reality–based simulation, a combination of both AR and VR, has been used in surgical training by producing three-dimensional printed models to isolate specific aspects of a surgical procedure.

INTRODUCTION

Imaging technologies are vital to the practice of modern spine surgery. This article presents a comprehensive review of the evolution of both invasive and noninvasive imaging technologies that are part of the arsenal of spinal diagnostics and surgical therapy. The text provides not only a historical lens to the evolution of the imaging technologies that are part of routine contemporary practice but also provides a detailed sketch of emerging technologies that are likely to become common in operating rooms in the next decade.

First-Generation Imaging Modalities

Radiographs

The use of radiographs for imaging bony structures of the spine can be dated back to at least 1897, when Cushing[1] published a case report on a patient with Brown-Sequard syndrome secondary to a gunshot injury (**Fig. 1**). Radiograph imaging of the spine was initially limited to the anterior-posterior plane, but by 1925 lateral views of the spine were able to be generated.[2] By the 1980s, there had been increasing interest in developing a robust radiographic definition of spinal instability using dynamic imaging (ie, flexion/extension views). In 1990, Boden and Wiesel[3] argued for the use of dynamic vertebral translation (defined as change in relative position between flexion and extension) rather than static displacement in evaluating spinal instability. The use of radiographs in this context continues to be a fixture in contemporary practice.

Disclosure: The authors have nothing to disclose.
Department of Neurosurgery, Cleveland Clinic Lerner College of Medicine of Case Western Reserve University, 9500 Euclid Avenue, Cleveland, OH 44106
* Corresponding author.
E-mail address: STEINM@CCF.ORG

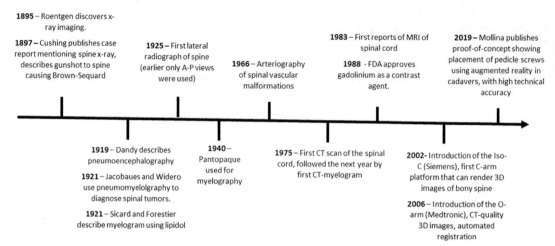

Fig. 1. Timeline showing the landmark events in the advancement of spinal imaging. 3D, three-dimensional; A-P, anteroposterior; CT, computed tomography; FDA, US Food and Drug Administration.

Myelography

Myelography (ie, radiographic imaging after injection of contrast into the subarachnoid space) was a major development in the early 1920s. Several contrast media were investigated, including air, oil-based preparations, and water-based media. In 1921, Dandy[4] published the use of pneumoencephalography to obtain an image of the brain, but remarked that the normal spinal cord could also been seen outlined by air. The same year, Jacobaeus and Wideroe used pneumomyelography to diagnose spinal tumors.[5,6] Sicard and Forestier[7] accidently injected Lipidol (an iodized poppy-seed oil) into the thecal sac and noticed that spinal structures could be visualized on radiographs. They developed the use of the technique through lumbar puncture and cisterna magna puncture. The early agents, including Lipidol and Pantopaque, had to be aspirated after radiography was complete, and were associated with a significant risk of arachnoiditis.[8] The contemporary agents, iohexol and iopamidol, arrived on the scene in the 1980s, and have been proved safe for routine use in practice.[9,10] Although not common, the technique of endomyelography has also been reported, wherein a cyst in the spinal cord is punctured, fluid is aspirated, air is injected, and radiographic images are obtained.[11] The utility of the procedure lies in its potential ability to identify vascular anomalies that could be a contraindication to surgery.

Vascular imaging

Imaging of vascular structures of the spinal cord was initially limited to visualization of the artery of Adamkiewicz and vascular malformations through injection of contrast into the

aorta or subclavian arteries.[8] With the popularization of the Seldinger technique, catheterization of the vertebral, intercostal, and lumbar arteries became popular, allowing more targeted imaging of vascular anatomy relevant to spinal surgery.[12] The next major milestone in vascular imaging came in the form of computer-generated angiograms based on contemporary three-dimensional (3D) imaging technologies (ie, computed tomography [CT]–based and MRI-based angiograms). These technologies served as preliminary guides before the gold standard catheter-based angiography could be performed to evaluate for a vascular malformation.

Three-Dimensional Imaging (Computed Tomography and MRI)

- CT. The start of 3D imaging of the spine occurred in the mid-1970s, when a CT scan was used to diagnose syringomyelia.[13] In 1976, the first reports of simultaneous intrathecal contrast injection and CT radiography (ie, CT myelogram) were reported.[14] Intravenous contrast soon became routine in clinical practice and was found to be an important application for perioperative spine imaging. There is great interest in distinguishing between extradural hypertrophic scar and reherniation of disc material in the postoperative period. In addition, it plays a valuable role in identifying bony destruction and remodeling in spine tumors and confirmation of instrumentation placement. Intravenous contrast–enhanced CT served as a possible tool for differentiating between various disorders and evaluating for infectious states.[15]

- MRI. In the 1980s, MRI became mainstream in clinical practice, offering superior image quality without exposure to radiation, but at the cost of being more time consuming and expensive. In 1988, the US Food and Drug Administration (FDA) approved gadolinium as a contrast agent, and gadolinium-enhanced MRI became an important part of the spine imaging arsenal.[16] The value of MRI in the assessment of soft tissue structures of the spine remains unsurpassed. Crisi and colleagues[17] were among the first to describe the enhancement of nerve roots, resulting from disc herniation. Although there is variability in estimates, there is consensus that MRI is a sensitive modality for disc morphology,[18] and intraobserver reliability is high for spondylolisthesis, facet arthropathy, and disc degeneration.[19] Some evidence does suggest that dynamic imaging (with patients undergoing axial loading in upright imaging systems and flexion/extension views) may change management in a small subset of patients (~2.5%), but supine MRI remains the mainstay.[20]

- Fetal imaging. MRI is now routinely used in the work-up of abnormal prenatal sonography of the spine, especially in the evaluation of neural tube defects.[21] Data suggest that MRI is an important adjunct to sonography because it provides information about topography, sac contents, and non–central nervous system findings. Importantly, MRI may lead to a change in management strategy in more than 20% of cases.[22]

- Magnetic resonance neurography imaging of individual nerves is possible through magnetic resonance neurography (MRN), which was reported in the late 1980s in cases of nerve entrapment in carpal tunnel syndrome.[23] However, the true value of MRN compared with sonography is in the imaging of deep nerves and smaller elements of major plexuses. For example, MRN is able to delineate individual elements of the brachial plexus and identify discrete disorders. Modern high-definition MRN is able to differentiate between neuromas in continuity and nerve discontinuities, allowing the identification of Sunderland grade 4 and 5 injuries respectively.[24]

- Diffusion-weighted imaging of the spine. Following experience of this imaging modality in the brain, diffusion-weighted imaging of the spinal cord was reported in 2000 and

technical developments have improved the technique in subsequent years.[25] Reports suggest exquisite sensitivity of this imaging modality for acute spinal cord ischemia, but it remains a largely underused technique in routine practice.[26]

The Integration of Imaging and Navigation

The 1990s saw important developments in image guidance in spine surgery.[27] Initially, there was interest in mirroring developments in cranial image-guided methods, which relied on either fiducial-based or surface-based registration methods to calibrate preoperative imaging with the anatomy of the patient during surgery. These registration methods proved challenging for spine because they were time consuming and at times inaccurate, and were soon supplanted by fluoroscopy-based navigation systems featuring a C-arm mobile fluoroscope.[28] Initially, these systems could not produce 3D reconstructions of bony anatomy and carried the risk of significant radiation exposure to surgical personnel. By 2002, a C-arm–based system was available on the market that could generate 3D reconstructions of the spine (Siremobil Iso-C 3D, Siemens Medical Solutions).[27] In 2006, the O-arm (Medtronic, Minneapolis, MN) was introduced and quickly became a distinct technology in the context of spinal surgery (**Fig. 2**). The O-arm could produce CT-quality images but eliminated the work-flow problems associated with the C-arm because of its breakable gantry, which allows lateral access to the patient. The O-arm also has autoregistration capability, which significantly reduced the time needed for navigation techniques. Modern O-arms are used in conjunction with navigation, creating a fully integrated image-guided surgery.

IMAGING FOR MINIMALLY INVASIVE SURGERY
High-Definition Endoscopes

Destandau and Foley[29] reported on the use of microendoscopes for spinal surgery in the late 1990s. The advantage of the endoscope compared with the operative microscope was the ability to see a wider range of the surgical field with a minimally invasive approach, but at the cost of nonstereoscopic vision and limited corridors for the manipulation of instruments.[30] As minimally invasive spine surgery developed to include both tubular and percutaneous approaches for a broad range of indications, the quality of endoscopic imaging also improved. Although early devices offered low-quality two-dimensional (2D) images,

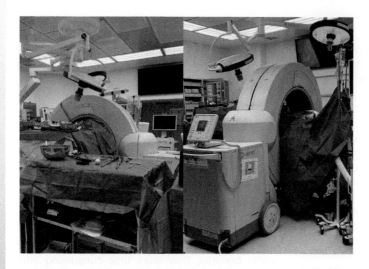

Fig. 2. Use of the O-arm (Medtronic, Minneapolis, MN) in spine surgery.

modern iterations of spinal endoscopes offer a high-definition (HD) or 4K image, with possible 3D capabilities based on either so-called insect-eye technology (ie, a single objective lens splits light along 2 paths then reconstructs a 3D image) or dual-optical technology.[31] For example, 3D neuroendoscopes have been reported to offer better depth perception without increasing operative time in the context of transsphenoidal surgery.[32] Many endoscope systems also allow for the use of visualization modes that permit real-time digital enhancement of the image based on preset optimized modes of illumination, contrast enhancement, and color shifting. In contrast with bulky operative microscopes, endoscopic imaging setups are usually limited to a single console and monitor, which significantly facilitates work flow in the operative room (**Fig. 3**).

Exoscopes

Advancements in imaging technology have led to the development of exoscopes, a camera system used outside the body, allowing projection of magnified, HD images to an external monitor. The focal distance is comparable with that of a standard microscope (~200–400 mm), allowing it to sit outside the body, unlike an endoscope, which has a much shorter focal length and requires placement directly adjacent to the surgical site (**Fig. 4**).[33] These systems work to bridge the gap between operative microscopes and endoscopes by combining the form factor of the endoscope with the image quality of the microscope. The current hope among adopters of this technology is mitigation of the limitations present in the standard operative microscope; namely, the cost of the device, its footprint within the operating room, the

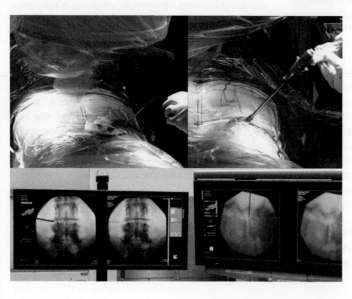

Fig. 3. Example of the use of the endoscope in spine surgery.

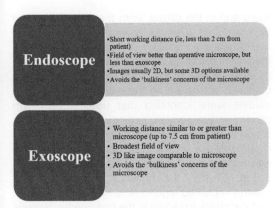

Endoscope
- Short working distance (ie, less than 2 cm from patient)
- Field of view better than operative microscope, but less than exoscope
- Images usually 2D, but some 3D options available
- Avoids the 'bulkiness' concerns of the microscope

Exoscope
- Working distance similar to or greater than microscope (up to 7.5 cm from patient)
- Broadest field of view
- 3D like image comparable to microscope
- Avoids the 'bulkiness' concerns of the microscope

Fig. 4. Comparing endoscope and exoscope.

complexity of use, the limited depth of field, and suboptimal ergonomics requiring the surgeon and assistant to bend their necks at uncomfortable angles for extended periods of time.

The use of the exoscope in spinal applications has been analyzed with a variety of different models used, including the 2D exoscope system (BrightMatter Servo, Synaptive Medical, and the Video Telescopic Monitor [VITOM], Karl Storz), the 3D exoscope system (VITOM-3D, Karl Storz), and the ORBEYE (Sony Olympus Medical Solutions, Inc.), which boasts 4K clarity alongside 3D technology. Use of 3D technology requires the surgeons to wear 3D glasses in order to create accurate stereopsis.

The exoscope is typically mounted on a robotic arm that holds the device over the surgical field while projecting the image to a monitor positioned in the line of sight of the surgeon and assistant. Newer iterations of the holders have integrated foot-pedal controllers and pilot devices that allow rapid and precise realignment of the exoscope. This setup allows a more natural positioning for the surgical team without the ergonomic demands often required to facilitate the optics of the operative microscope. In addition, the surgical view provided by the exoscope is shared by all members of the operating room team without the degradation in quality that may be present when using accessory optics. In contrast, video captured by the microscope that is projected to external monitors in the operating room may be off-center or of significantly lower quality, which impairs nonsurgeon visualization. As such, the exoscope acts as a useful educational adjunct, aiding in the training of residents, fellows, and nurses alike.

Several studies have directly compared the exoscope with the operative microscope in both cadaveric and clinical spinal surgeries. Kwan and colleagues[34] used the ORBEYE system (3D 4K-HD) during 10 spinal surgery cases, including anterior cervical discectomy and instrumented

fusions (ACDFs), cervical laminectomies, cervical corpectomy, and lumbar laminectomies. Identified advantages included improved ergonomics, the ability to switch between loupe and 3D magnification instantly, and educational benefits from a shared operative view. Disadvantages included increased scope adjustments and a trend toward increased operative time; however, the investigators thought that this would be mitigated with greater experience with the technology. Moisi and colleagues[35] compared the microscope with the exoscope (the 2D Synaptive BrightMatter Servo) in grading cadaveric lumbar laminotomies performed by senior neurosurgical residents and fellows. Data regarding the duration of the procedure with blinded grading of quality of decompression and presence of complications were collected and no significant difference was identified in any domain. The exoscope was praised for its improved ergonomics, teaching potential, and increased depth of field (which reduced the amount of refocusing required), whereas its lack of stereoscopy was a noted limitation. Shirzadi and colleagues[36] conducted a prospective cohort study in which the VITOM system was used in single-level and 2-level lumbar decompressions as well as transforaminal interbody fusions with the operative microscope acting as control. No significant difference was identified in the operative time or postoperative hospital stay between the two 24-patient cohorts, and no intraoperative complications were encountered in either group. Identified advantages included ergonomics, cost, teaching benefits, portability/decreased weight, and improved depth of field. Disadvantages included lack of stereopsis, which was deemed minimal as surgeon experience with the technology increased, and difficulty with VITOM repositioning, which was considered to be significantly mitigated with introduction of a hydraulic scope holder. Mamelak and colleagues[37] reinforced these findings in a study using the VITOM that contained 6 spinal procedures including lumbar laminotomies/foraminotomies and anterior cervical discectomies, stating that the technology "even in its current configuration, is suited for almost all spinal surgeries," although criticism was again levied against the cumbersome nature of the pneumatic holder of the exoscope. A study by Oertel and Burkhardt[38] included 11 spinal procedures performed with the VITOM-3D. The study reinforced the equality of image quality, illumination, and depth perception to that of the microscope, and praised the excellent mobility and ease of repositioning. Overall, they found that the technology was "an excellent alternative for the treatment of degenerative spinal pathologies."

Although more clinical trials would be required to objectively determine the exoscope's benefits and detriments, current literature seems to clearly outline its perceived advantages and its limitations in spinal surgery applications. Although it may not completely replace the operative microscope's proven utility and reliability at this point in time, the cost, ergonomics, and uniform visualization benefits of the exoscope are attractive, especially at teaching hospitals. The legitimate concerns against the endoscope seem to have remedies under development. The lack of stereopsis was answered with the introduction of 3D exoscopes and, with continued research and development, satisfactory holders should further quell complaints about the difficulty in repositioning and refocusing the device.

THE AGE OF AUGMENTED VISUALIZATION

Augmented reality (AR), defined as adding digital elements to a live view by using a camera, is an emerging imaging technology in spine surgery (**Fig. 5**). In addition, virtual reality (VR) and mixed reality (MR) are also gaining acceptance. VR is a complete immersive experience that shuts out the physical world (eg, Oculus Rift). MR combines elements of VR and AR to produce a real world in which digital objects interact (eg, Microsoft's HoloLens).

There are 2 main types of AR: marker based and markerless. Marker-based AR uses fiducial markers and image recognition to identify objects. When the camera feed detects a marker (ie, QR code), the device compares the information with markers in its database until finding a match, thereby displaying the AR image. Markerless AR has no preprogrammed images on the device, purely using patterns, colors, or other features for recognition.

Surgeons have been eager to find ways to incorporate AR into their practice both in the operating

room and in the clinics. With the development of Google Glass (Google, Mountain View, CA) the use of heads-up displays in medicine has accelerated. Multiple studies have shown the rapid transmission of information with AR and heads-up displays. In a review by Yoon and colleagues,[39] 5 studies were identified that used a heads-up display in live surgical settings and 5 studies in which it was used for simulation. The technology is primarily used in cranial surgeries and for live image capture and streaming for educational purposes. Chiefly, the benefits of heads-up AR include improved ergonomics, multitasking ability, and the ability to record in the first person. Various drawbacks include asthenopia caused by the small projection, the battery life of the device, and patient privacy. In addition to heads-up display, AR is increasingly being used to assist in placement of instrumentation in spine surgery. The improvement in 3D visualization and graphics has increased clinicians' reliance on image guidance. Early adopters of AR in spine have used it in low-risk procedures, such as bone biopsies, spinal injections, and other MRI-based interventions.[40–42]

Molina and colleagues[43] studied the use of AR-assisted pedicle screws on a cadaveric model. Their goal was to evaluate the accuracy of AR-assisted pedicle screw insertion compared with conventional insertion techniques. Their results showed superiority when comparing AR with freehand insertion, and noninferiority when comparing AR with robotics-assisted computer navigated and manual computer navigated insertion. This technique has also been tested on thoracic pedicle screws, which are known to be more challenging than lumbar pedicle screws. Luciano and colleagues[44] used an AR-based simulator with haptic feedback. They found 15% mean score improvement and a greater than 50% reduction in standard from practice session to test session. This finding has also been replicated in a cadaveric study by Elmi-Terander and colleagues,[45] finding superiority of AR compared with freehand technique regarding overall accuracy (85% vs 64%; $P<.05$) and reduction in breaches beyond 4 mm (2% vs 25%; $P<.05$).

The use of intraoperative CT (iCT) in operating rooms is becoming more routine. Typically, after the dorsal spine is exposed, an iCT scan is obtained and registered to an AR-based reference system. This system can be integrated with BrainLab (BrainLab AG, Munich, Germany), Stryker (Stryker, Kalamazoo, MI), or Medtronic (Medtronic, Minneapolis, MN) navigation systems. There are also systems such as the 7D Surgical (7D Surgical, Toronto, Canada) that use a preoperative CT scan and then use flash registration to navigate intraoperatively (**Fig. 6**). The accuracy of AR surgical

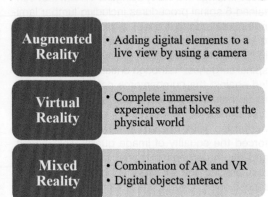

Fig. 5. Comparison of the different types of AR.

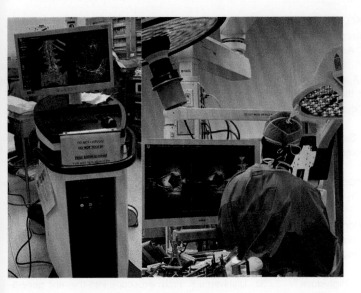

Fig. 6. Example of the use of AR in spine surgery with the 7D Surgical (Toronto, Canada) image guidance system.

navigation was confirmed by Burstrom and colleagues[46] in their cadaveric study. The technical accuracy of pedicle screw placement was 1.7 mm at bone entry point with an angular deviation of 1.7° in the axial and 1.6° in the sagittal plane with no additional use of ionizing radiation. The amount of radiation exposure from iCT is kept minimal through the use of low-dose protocols (0.35–0.98 mSv for cervical, 2.16–6.92 mSv for thoracic, and 3.55–4.20 mSv for lumbar surgeries).[47]

VR-based simulators are being used in surgical education across multiple disciplines. Spine surgeons are using these stimulators to become facile in the technical nuances of various procedures, such as pedicle screw placement, vertebroplasty, and facet joint injection.[48]

MR-based simulation, a combination of both AR and VR, is slowly establishing a presence in surgical training. Bova and colleagues[49] have used 3D printing to manufacture physical models based on deidentified patient data. These data have then been presented as surgical challenges for residents in training, allowing individuals to focus on specific areas of deficiency.

SUMMARY

Society has come a long way from the days of the experimental method and exploratory surgery. With the use of AR, VR, and MR, preparation for surgery and the integration of new technologies have been improved to a new standard. These modalities provide excellent case-specific training modules to break down each step of an operation in isolation. The goal of providers is to understand how to find this harmonious balance and effectively use this quintessential resource to enhance patient care and surgical training.

REFERENCES

1. Cushing H. Haematomyelia from gunshot wound of the cervical spine. Bull Johns Hopkins Hosp 1897; 8:195–7.
2. Emch TM, Modic MT. Imaging of lumbar degenerative disk disease: history and current state. Skeletal Radiol 2011;40(9):1175.
3. Boden SD, Wiesel SW. Lumbosacral segmental motion in normal individuals. Have we been measuring instability properly? Spine 1990;15(6): 571–6.
4. Dandy WE. Roentgenography of the brain after the injection of air into the spinal canal. Ann Surg 1919;70(4):397.
5. Jacobaeus H. On insuffiation of air into the spinal canal for diagnostic purposes in cases of tumors in the spinal canal. Acta Med Scand 1921;55(1):555–64.
6. Wideroe S. Über die diagnostische Bedeutung der intraspinalen Luftinjektionen bei Rückenmarksleiden, besonders bei Geschwülsten. Z. Chir 1921; 48:394–7.
7. Forestier S. Methode generale d'exploration radiologique par l'huile iodee (Lipiodol). Bull Mem Soc Med Hop Paris 1922;463–8.
8. Hoeffner E, Mukherji S, Srinivasan A, et al. Neuroradiology back to the future: spine imaging. AJNR Am J Neuroradiol 2012;33(6):999–1006.
9. Eldevik OP, Nakstad P, Kendall BE, et al. Iohexol in lumbar myelography: preliminary results from an open, noncomparative multicenter clinical study. AJNR Am J Neuroradiol 1983;4(3):299–301.

10. Witwer G, Cacayorin ED, Bernstein AD, et al. Iopamidol and metrizamide for myelography: prospective double-blind clinical trial. AJR Am J Roentgenol 1984;143(4):869–73.

11. Dietemann J, Babin E, Wackenheim A, et al. Percutaneous puncture of spinal cysts in the diagnosis and therapy of syringomyelia and cystic tumors. Neuroradiology 1982;24(1):59–63.

12. Di Criro G, Doppman J, Ommaya AK. Selective arteriography of arteriovenous aneurysms of spinal cord. Radiology 1967;88(6):1065–77.

13. Di Chiro G, Axelbaum SP, Schellinger D, et al. Computerized axial tomography in syringomyelia. N Engl J Med 1975;292(1):13–6.

14. Di Chiro G, Schellinger D. Computed tomography of spinal cord after lumbar intrathecal introduction of metrizamide (computer-assisted myelography). Radiology 1976;120(1):101–4.

15. Yang PJ, Seeger JF, Dzioba RB, et al. High-dose iv contrast in CT scanning of the postoperative lumbar spine. AJNR Am J Neuroradiol 1986;7(4):703–7.

16. Hueftle M, Modic M, Ross J, et al. Lumbar spine: postoperative MR imaging with Gd-DTPA. Radiology 1988;167(3):817–24.

17. Crisi G, Carpeggiani P, Trevisan C. Gadolinium-enhanced nerve roots in lumbar disk herniation. AJNR Am J Neuroradiol 1993;14(6):1379–92.

18. Jarvik JG, Deyo RA. Diagnostic evaluation of low back pain with emphasis on imaging. Ann Intern Med 2002;137(7):586–97.

19. Arana E, Royuela A, Kovacs FM, et al. Lumbar spine: agreement in the interpretation of 1.5-T MR images by using the Nordic Modic Consensus Group classification form. Radiology 2010;254(3):809–17.

20. Hiwatashi A, Danielson B, Moritani T, et al. Axial loading during MR imaging can influence treatment decision for symptomatic spinal stenosis. AJNR Am J Neuroradiol 2004;25(2):170–4.

21. Glenn O, Barkovich A. Magnetic resonance imaging of the fetal brain and spine: an increasingly important tool in prenatal diagnosis, part 1. AJNR Am J Neuroradiol 2006;27(8):1604–11.

22. Saleem SN, Said A-H, Abdel-Raouf M, et al. Fetal MRI in the evaluation of fetuses referred for sonographically suspected neural tube defects (NTDs): impact on diagnosis and management decision. Neuroradiology 2009;51(11):761–72.

23. Middleton W, Kneeland J, Kellman G, et al. MR imaging of the carpal tunnel: normal anatomy and preliminary findings in the carpal tunnel syndrome. AJR Am J Roentgenol 1987;148(2):307–16.

24. Chhabra A, Andreisek G, Soldatos T, et al. MR neurography: past, present, and future. AJR Am J Roentgenol 2011;197(3):583–91.

25. Bammer R, Fazekas F, Augustin M, et al. Diffusion-weighted MR imaging of the spinal cord. AJNR Am J Neuroradiol 2000;21(3):587–91.

26. Thurnher MM, Bammer R. Diffusion-weighted MR imaging (DWI) in spinal cord ischemia. Neuroradiology 2006;48(11):795–801.

27. Helm PA, Teichman R, Hartmann SL, et al. Spinal navigation and imaging: history, trends, and future. IEEE Trans Med Imaging 2015;34(8):1738–46.

28. Nottmeier EW, Crosby TL. Timing of paired points and surface matching registration in three-dimensional (3D) image-guided spinal surgery. Clin Spine Surg 2007;20(4):268–70.

29. Smith MM, Foley KT. Microendoscopic discectomy (MED): the first 100 cases. Neurosurgery 1988; 43(3):702.

30. Ricciardi L, Chaichana KL, Cardia A, et al. The exoscope in neurosurgery: an innovative "point of view". A systematic review of the technical, surgical, and educational aspects. World Neurosurg 2019;124: 136–44.

31. Nishiyama K. From exoscope into the next generation. J Korean Neurosurg Soc 2017;60(3):289–93.

32. Tabaee A, Anand VK, Fraser JF, et al. Three-dimensional endoscopic pituitary surgery. Neurosurgery 2009;64(5 Suppl 2):288–93 [discussion: 294–5].

33. Mamelak AN, Nobuto T, Berci G. Initial clinical experience with a high-definition exoscope system for microneurosurgery. Neurosurgery 2010;67(2):476–83.

34. Kwan K, Schneider JR, Du V, et al. Lessons learned using a high-definition 3-dimensional exoscope for spinal surgery. Oper Neurosurg (Hagerstown) 2019;16(5):619–25.

35. Moisi MD, Hoang K, Tubbs RS, et al. Advancement of surgical visualization methods: comparison study between traditional microscopic surgery and a novel robotic optoelectronic visualization tool for spinal surgery. World Neurosurg 2017;98:273–7.

36. Shirzadi A, Mukherjee D, Drazin DG, et al. Use of the video telescope operating monitor (VITOM) as an alternative to the operating microscope in spine surgery. Spine 2012;37(24):E1517–23.

37. Mamelak AN, Danielpour M, Black KL, et al. A high-definition exoscope system for neurosurgery and other microsurgical disciplines: preliminary report. Surg Innov 2008;15(1):38–46.

38. Oertel JM, Burkhardt BW. Vitom-3D for exoscopic neurosurgery: initial experience in cranial and spinal procedures. World Neurosurg 2017;105:153–62.

39. Yoon JW, Chen RE, Kim EJ, et al. Augmented reality for the surgeon: systematic review. Int J Med Robot 2018;14(4):e1914.

40. George S, Kesavadas T. Low cost augmented reality for training of MRI-guided needle biopsy of the spine. Stud Health Technol Inform 2008;132: 138–40.

41. Weiss CR, Marker DR, Fischer GS, et al. Augmented reality visualization using Image-Overlay for MR-guided interventions: system description, feasibility,

and initial evaluation in a spine phantom. AJR Am J Roentgenol 2011;196(3):W305–7.

42. Fritz J, U-Thainual P, Ungi T, et al. Augmented reality visualization with image overlay for MRI-guided intervention: accuracy for lumbar spinal procedures with a 1.5-T MRI system. AJR Am J Roentgenol 2012;198(3):W266–73.

43. Molina CA, Theodore N, Ahmed AK, et al. Augmented reality-assisted pedicle screw insertion: a cadaveric proof-of-concept study. J Neurosurg Spine 2019;1–8.

44. Luciano CJ, Banerjee PP, Bellotte B, et al. Learning retention of thoracic pedicle screw placement using a high-resolution augmented reality simulator with haptic feedback. Neurosurgery 2011;69(1 Suppl Operative):ons14–9 [discussion: ons14-19].

45. Elmi-Terander A, Skulason H, Soderman M, et al. Surgical navigation technology based on augmented reality and integrated 3D intraoperative imaging: a spine cadaveric feasibility and accuracy study. Spine (Phila Pa 1976) 2016;41(21): E1303–11.

46. Burstrom G, Nachabe R, Persson O, et al. Augmented and virtual reality instrument tracking for minimally invasive spine surgery: a feasibility and accuracy study. Spine (Phila Pa 1976) 2019; 44(15):1097–104.

47. Carl B, Bopp M, Sass B, et al. Implementation of augmented reality support in spine surgery. Eur Spine J 2019;28(7):1697–711.

48. Pfandler M, Lazarovici M, Stefan P, et al. Virtual reality-based simulators for spine surgery: a systematic review. Spine J 2017;17(9):1352–63.

49. Bova FJ, Rajon DA, Friedman WA, et al. Mixed-reality simulation for neurosurgical procedures. Neurosurgery 2013;73(Suppl 1):138–45.

Robotic-Assisted Spinal Surgery
Current Generation Instrumentation and New Applications

Clay M. Elswick, MD[a], Michael J. Strong, MD, PhD, MPH[a],
Jacob R. Joseph, MD[a], Yamaan Saadeh, MD[a], Mark Oppenlander, MD[a],
Paul Park, MD[b],*

KEYWORDS

• Pedicle screw • Navigation • Robotics • Spine • Image guidance

KEY POINTS

• Robotics in spinal surgery is still relatively new and primarily used for pedicle screw placement but has the potential to impact other aspects of spinal surgery.
• Robotic-assisted pedicle screw placement is accurate.
• Robotic-assisted instrumentation can reduce radiation exposure to the surgeon and operating room staff.
• Current-generation robots have the capacity for navigation, which, although elementary at this stage, can aid in localization and trajectory planning, positively impacting retractor placement in minimally invasive procedures, assessing extent of decompression, and assisting cage placement.

INTRODUCTION

The promise of robotics in surgery is to increase efficiency, increase consistency, and reduce human error, leading to improved outcomes. Although robotics is relatively new to spinal surgery, in other surgical fields, there is a suggestion that use of a surgical robot is becoming the standard of care.[1] The first reported use of a robot in neurosurgery dates to 1988[2] and involved a robotic-assisted brain biopsy.[2] The introduction of a robot into spinal surgery, however, did not occur until the mid-2000s, with the first reports published in 2016.[3,4]

The initial impetus to apply robotics in spinal surgery was the relatively high rate of suboptimal pedicle screw placement by freehand technique and fluoroscopic guidance.[5] Consequently, the first generation of spinal robots was designed for pedicle screw placement and consisted of a frame-based rigid drill guide for insertion of Kirschner wires (K-wires). Subsequent iterations have obviated the need for K-wire usage for pedicle screw placement. Beyond increased accuracy, another benefit of the use of spinal robotics is reduced radiation exposure to the surgeon and operating room staff.

Presently, spinal robots can consistently place pedicle screws with high accuracy.[6] Consequently, there has been a focus on adding features to potentially impact other aspects of surgery

Disclosure Statement: Dr P. Park is a consultant for Medtronic, Globus Medical, NuVasive, and Zimmer Biomet; receives royalties from Globus Medical; and receives non–study-related clinical/research support from Pfizer and Vertex (Boston, MA, USA). The author authors have nothing to disclose.

[a] Department of Neurosurgery, University of Michigan, 3552 Taubman Center, Box, 0338, 1500 East Medical Center Drive, Ann Arbor, MI 48109, USA; [b] Neurological Surgery, Department of Neurosurgery, University of Michigan, 3552 Taubman Center, Box 0338, 1500 East Medical Center Drive, Ann Arbor, MI 48109, USA
* Corresponding author.
E-mail address: ppark@med.umich.edu

beyond pedicle screw placement. One new feature is the ability to use freehand navigation. In this study, we review the surgical technique, including use of navigation and outcomes, for the recently introduced Excelsius GPS robot (Globus Medical, Inc., Audubon, PA).

METHODS

Institutional review board approval was obtained for this study. The medical records and imaging data were reviewed. Twenty-eight patients who underwent placement of pedicle screw instrumentation with the Excelsius GPS robot from February 2018 to March 2019 were identified for the analysis. Data recorded consisted of demographic and surgical characteristics and such variables as patient age, gender, body mass index, diagnosis, and levels treated.

Pedicle Screw Insertion Accuracy

All patients had postprocedure computed tomography (CT) imaging that was analyzed for accuracy of pedicle screw placement. A modified Gertzbein-Robbins scale (GRS) was used to calculate accuracy. The original GRS measured pedicle screw accuracy in the axial plane only.[7] We modified the GRS by analyzing screw placement in the sagittal and coronal planes, as well as the axial plane, for increased sensitivity for pedicle screw breach (**Fig. 1**). The same grading of the original

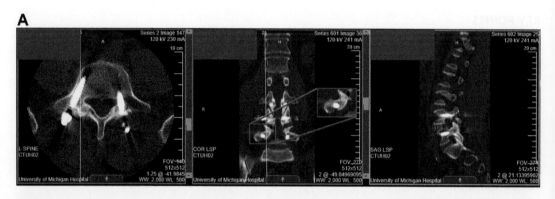

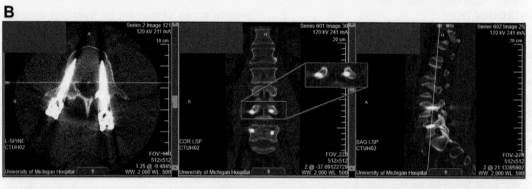

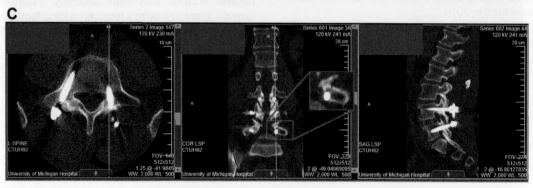

Fig. 1. Examples of pedicle screw breaches in 3 patients (A–C) found on multiplanar CT imaging.

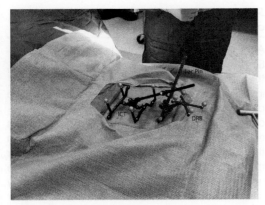

Fig. 2. Placement of iliac pin, DRB, and ICT registration frame for acquisition of ICT. On completion of image acquisition, the ICT is removed.

GRS was maintained. GRS A constituted a pedicle screw contained entirely within the pedicle; GRS B constituted a breach of the pedicle measuring 0 to 2 mm; GRS C constituted a breach measuring 2 to 4 mm; GRS D represented a breach measuring 4 to 6 mm; and GRS E represented a breach of greater than 6 mm. CT imaging was reviewed by 2 authors (MJS and CME).

Surgical Technique: Robotic-Assisted Pedicle Screw Placement

The patient is positioned prone on a radiolucent frame, prepped, and draped widely in the standard manner. Subsequent steps differ for a minimally invasive versus open procedure. For a minimally invasive procedure, a small incision is made overlying the inferior aspect of the posterior superior iliac spine. An iliac pin is impacted into the bone. A dynamic reference base (DRB) is then attached to the iliac pin. The next step depends on whether preoperative CT or intraoperative CT (ICT) is used. For preoperative CT, a standard fluoroscope with a specialized registration attachment is used to merge the preoperative CT data with the target spinal segments. For ICT, an ICT registration frame is also attached to the iliac pin (**Fig. 2**). The frame is removed after ICT acquisition. For an open procedure, exposure of the spine is first performed and then a spinous process clamp is placed. The DRB is attached to the spinous process clamp. For ICT acquisition, the ICT frame is also attached.

Attention is then turned to pedicle screw planning. Using the planning software, the optimal trajectory, size, and length of each pedicle screw is determined (**Fig. 3**). The spinal robot is then draped and positioned in the surgical field. For a minimally invasive procedure, the robot arm and end effector tube are positioned over the skin according to the screw plans to determine the incision sites. After localization of the paramedian incision sites, an incision is made, and the underlying fascia is opened longitudinally with Bovie cautery. A lengthy opening of the fascia allows

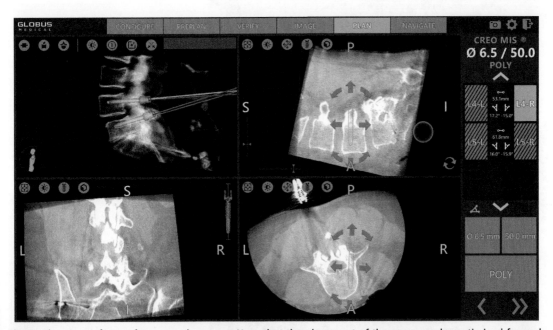

Fig. 3. Planning software for screw placement. Note that the placement of the screw can be optimized for each pedicle in terms of trajectory (*arrows* allow fine adjustment), length, and diameter of screw. The panel in the upper left shows a 3-dimensional overview of the planned screws.

unimpeded passage of the instruments. Each of the navigated instruments (ie, drill, tap, and screwdriver) is inserted through the robot end effector tube. For an open procedure, typically a wide exposure is necessary to allow passage of the instruments, given that planned screw trajectories are more idealized, resulting in a more triangulated direction. Alternatively, the screws can be inserted in a transmuscular manner. After appropriate exposure, the robotic arm automatically positions itself according to each screw plan. The drill is inserted with the end effector tube rigidly maintaining the appropriate trajectory (**Fig. 4**). Note that the drill is navigated so that the surgeon can track the drill as it traverses the pedicle in real time. Once the pedicle screw tract is drilled, a navigated tap is used, followed by insertion of the appropriate screw. In the case of a minimally invasive procedure, the screw is attached to screw extenders before insertion.

Surgical Technique: Navigation Applications of the Robot

After the pedicle screws are inserted, the navigation capability of the robot can be used. Presently, the navigation options are limited to use of a navigation pointer; however, use of a navigation pointer can positively impact aspects of the procedure, particularly in minimally invasive cases resulting in decreased need for fluoroscopy. In the case of minimally invasive surgery (MIS) for transforaminal lumbar interbody fusion (TLIF), the navigation pointer is used to determine the entry site for the initial dilator used for tubular retractor placement (**Fig. 5**A). After dilation and tubular retractor placement, the navigation pointer can confirm appropriate placement overlying the facet and lateral lamina and confirm adequate trajectory (**Fig. 5**B). In the case of an MIS laminectomy, the navigated pointer can assist in determining the adequacy of contralateral decompression (**Fig. 6**).

Fig. 4. The end effector tube is positioned according to the screw plan with navigated drill.

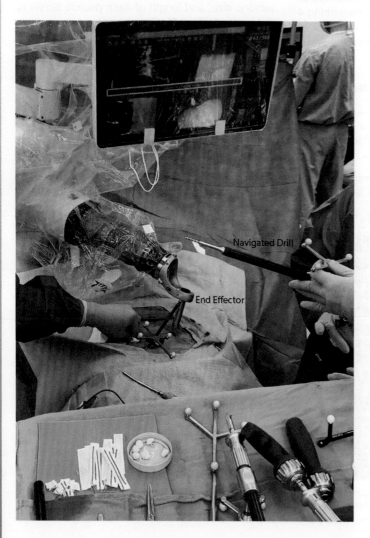

The trajectory view afforded by the navigated pointer also can assist in determining cage placement during MIS TLIF (**Fig. 7**).

Statistical Analysis

Descriptive statistics are reported for the cohort with mean and standard deviation (SD) for continuous variables and proportions for dichotomous and categorical variables. Excel (Microsoft, Redmond, WA) was used for the analysis.

RESULTS

Of the 28 patients, 16 (57.1%) were men, 12 (42.9%) were women, and the mean age of the

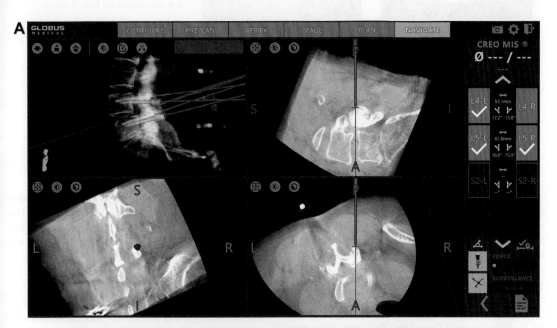

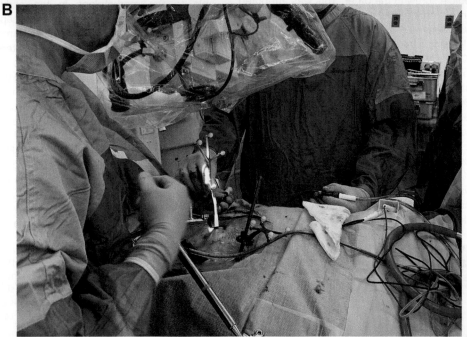

Fig. 5. (*A*) Use of the navigation pointer to determine location and trajectory for tubular retractor placement. (*B*) Tubular retractor is positioned for minimally invasive TLIF. The navigation pointer is used to confirm appropriate tubular retractor placement orthogonal to disc space and over the facet and lateral lamina.

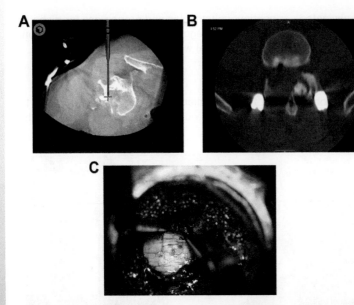

Fig. 6. (*A*) Navigation pointer in the contralateral spinal canal confirming adequate decompression for the minimally invasive unilateral approach for bilateral decompression. (*B*) Postoperative axial CT image shows adequate bilateral decompression from unilateral approach. (*C*) Navigation pointer in the contralateral spinal canal.

cohort was 61.5 years (**Table 1**). The average body mass index was 30.8. The most common diagnoses included spondylolisthesis (53.6%) and degenerative disease with stenosis (21.4%). A total of 127 screws were placed with robotic assistance. On evaluation with fluoroscopy, 2 (1.6%) screws were noted to be outside the pedicle. Both occurred during an MIS TLIF and involved the left L5 pedicle screw in one case and the left S1 pedicle screw in the other. This was attributed to skiving during the drilling process. These 2 screws were removed and inserted into the pedicle using a traditional percutaneous technique with K-wire placement and fluoroscopic guidance.

A total of 125 screws were evaluated with postoperative CT to determine accuracy. Of these, 104 (83.2%) screws were classified as GRS A, and 18 (14.4%) screws were classified as GRS B. Three of 125 screws (2.4%) were classified as GRS C.

The most frequent levels treated were L5 (17.3%), S1 (11%), and L4 (9.4% on right and 10.2% on left). Of the 21 non-GRS A pedicle screws, 6 were placed at L3 (3 on the right and 3 on the left), which represented 33.3% of the pedicle screws placed at that level. The next

highest percentage of non-GRS A pedicle screws were at L5, with 6 on the right side and 5 on the left side (27.3% and 22.7%, respectively). Of the 3 GRS-C pedicle screws, 2 occurred at the left L5 pedicle and the other at the right L3 pedicle.

DISCUSSION

The first iterations of the spine robot became available to the marketplace in the early 2000s. Although they did not have navigation capabilities, they did facilitate pedicle screw placement. One such robot that has been studied extensively is the SpineAssist (MAZOR Robotics Inc., Orlando, FL). Molliqaj and colleagues[8] published their retrospective review in 2017 and found that 83% of their screws placed with robot assistance were classified as GRS A. Another 10% were GRS B. In their comparative series, 76% of fluoroscopically placed screws were placed with GRS A accuracy. Another 12.9% of the fluoroscopically placed screws were GRS B. The investigators found that the proportion of accurate pedicle screws (defined as GRS A and B) were statistically higher in the robot-assisted group than the freehand

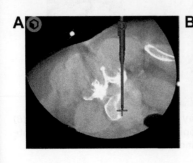 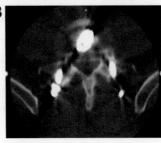

Fig. 7. (*A*) The navigation pointer within the disc space that is the planned placement of the cage. (*B*) Postoperative axial CT shows that the interbody cage is positioned according to the trajectory of the navigation pointer.

Table 1
Summary of demographics, clinical history, and surgical characteristics

	n = 28
Demographics and Clinical History	
Age, mean y (SD)	61.5 (12.1)
Gender, n (%)	
Male	16 (57.1)
Female	12 (42.9)
Body mass index, mean (SD)	30.8 (5.7)
Spondylolisthesis	15 (53.6)
Deformity	5 (17.9)
Degenerative disease with stenosis	6 (21.4)
Other[a]	2 (7.1)
Surgical characteristics	
Total screws placed, n	127
Total screws evaluated with CT, n	125
GRS A, n (%)	104 (83.2)
GRS B, n (%)	18 (14.4)
GRS C, n (%)	3 (2.4)
GRS D, n (%)	0 (0)
GRS E, n (%)	2 (1.6)[b]

Level, n (%)	Right		Left	
	Screws Placed	Misplaced[c]	Screws Placed	Misplaced[c]
T12	1 (0.8)	0 (0)	1 (0.8)	0 (0)
L1	2 (1.6)	0 (0)	2 (1.6)	0 (0)
L2	3 (2.4)	0 (0)	3 (2.4)	0 (0)
L3	9 (7.1)	0 (0)	9 (7.1)	1 (11.1)
L4	12 (9.4)	0 (0)	13 (10.2)	0 (0)
L5	22 (17.3)	0 (0)	22 (17.3)	3 (13.6)
S1	14 (11.0)	0 (0)	14 (11.0)	1 (7.1)

[a] Other includes osteolysis with fracture and flat back syndrome.
[b] The 2 screws that were classified as GRS E were determined intraoperatively without formal measurements in multiplanes; because it was determined that these screws were out of the pedicle, we arbitrarily classified them as GRS E.
[c] Misplaced includes all screws GRS C–E.

fluoroscopy group. A number of other studies have also corroborated the use of the SpineAssist and demonstrated its safety,[9,10] and, in some cases, its superiority.[11] Conversely, Ringel and colleagues[12] found superior accuracy with traditional freehand placement as compared with robotic-assisted placement, with accuracy of 93% by freehand and 85% with robot assistance. The newer-generation Mazor X robot has also demonstrated favorable results. In a single-institution retrospective study comparing the Mazor X with traditional CT-based navigation, Khan and colleagues[13] found comparable results with high pedicle screw accuracy (189/190 screws with Ravi grade I accuracy by robotic assistance and 157/165 Ravi grade

I accuracy by 3D-CT navigation) but improved fluoroscopy time and time-per-screw placement.

The Excelsius GPS robot (Globus Medical) gained US Food and Drug Administration approval in 2017. Formal studies demonstrating the accuracy of the Excelsius GPS robot have not been previously published, but Zygourakis and colleagues[14] published a case report in July 2018 demonstrating its use in a revision lumbar decompression and fusion. This study marks one of the first series analyzing the use of the Excelsius GPS robot, and the accuracy of the robot presented here (GRS A 83.2%, GRS B 14.4%) is in line with previous published series that documented accuracy with spinal robotics.[8,13]

Two (1.6%) of the robotic-assisted screws missed the pedicle completely, which required revision using traditional percutaneous fluoroscopic technique. This type of inaccuracy has been described previously and we feel it was most likely due to skiving of the drill due to an irregularity of the bone surface morphology, as can occur with facet arthropathy.[6] Since these 2 cases, we have taken care to plan a slightly more medial trajectory if the entry site for the pedicle screw is on a sloped surface. Soft tissue resistance has also been described as a mechanism for inaccuracy due to the inability to obtain a medialized trajectory. This was less likely an issue in our 2 cases, as they involved paramedian approach for the MIS TLIF.

Another proposed benefit of spinal robotics is the reduced radiation exposure to the surgeon and surgical team. Numerous studies have demonstrated the dramatic amount of ionizing radiation that the spine surgeon receives during a lumbar fusion operation.[15] Use of a spinal robot in lieu of fluoroscopy largely negates these high doses of radiation.

Another advantage of the current generation of spinal robots as compared with the early generation is the capacity for navigation, which can impact other aspects of the procedure beyond screw placement. Although the navigation capability afforded by the current robot is elementary, the navigation pointer can be used to determine location and trajectory, which are most beneficial for minimally invasive procedures, such as the MIS TLIF shown in this study. This can reduce the amount of radiation exposure to the surgeon and staff. It is our opinion that future generations of this robot will likely expand the navigation capabilities to more effectively impact decompression, disc space preparation, and cage placement.

SUMMARY

The Excelsius GPS robot can accurately place pedicle screws, with accuracy comparable to other spinal robotic systems. The capacity for navigation is a benefit of the present version of the spinal robot that can positively impact portions of the procedure beyond screw placement. Given that the current generation of the spinal robot can effectively place pedicle screws, future iterations of the device will enhance other aspects of spinal surgery.

REFERENCES

1. Lane T. A short history of robotic surgery. Ann R Coll Surg Engl 2018;100(6_sup):5–7.
2. Kwoh YS, Hou J, Jonckheere EA, et al. A robot with improved absolute positioning accuracy for CT guided stereotactic brain surgery. IEEE Trans Biomed Eng 1988;35(2):153–60.
3. Sukovich W, Brink-Danan S, Hardenbrook M. Miniature robotic guidance for pedicle screw placement in posterior spinal fusion: early clinical experience with the SpineAssist. Int J Med Robot 2006;2(2):114–22.
4. Barzilay Y, Liebergall M, Fridlander A, et al. Miniature robotic guidance for spine surgery–introduction of a novel system and analysis of challenges encountered during the clinical development phase at two spine centres. Int J Med Robot 2006;2(2):146–53.
5. Ghasem A, Sharma A, Greif DN, et al. The arrival of robotics in spine surgery: a review of the literature. Spine (Phila Pa 1976) 2018;43(23):1670–7.
6. Joseph JR, Smith BW, Liu X, et al. Current applications of robotics in spine surgery: a systematic review of the literature. Neurosurg Focus 2017;42(5):E2.
7. Gertzbein SD, Robbins SE. Accuracy of pedicular screw placement in vivo. Spine (Phila Pa 1976) 1990;15(1):11–4.
8. Molliqaj G, Schatlo B, Alaid A, et al. Accuracy of robot-guided versus freehand fluoroscopy-assisted pedicle screw insertion in thoracolumbar spinal surgery. Neurosurg Focus 2017;42(5):E14.
9. Pechlivanis I, Kiriyanthan G, Engelhardt M, et al. Percutaneous placement of pedicle screws in the lumbar spine using a bone mounted miniature robotic system: first experiences and accuracy of screw placement. Spine (Phila Pa 1976) 2009;34(4):392–8.
10. Devito DP, Kaplan L, Dietl R, et al. Clinical acceptance and accuracy assessment of spinal implants guided with SpineAssist surgical robot: retrospective study. Spine (Phila Pa 1976) 2010;35(24):2109–15.
11. Kantelhardt SR, Martinez R, Baerwinkel S, et al. Perioperative course and accuracy of screw positioning in conventional, open robotic-guided and percutaneous robotic-guided, pedicle screw placement. Eur Spine J 2011;20(6):860–8.
12. Ringel F, Stuer C, Reinke A, et al. Accuracy of robot-assisted placement of lumbar and sacral pedicle screws: a prospective randomized comparison to conventional freehand screw implantation. Spine (Phila Pa 1976) 2012;37(8):E496–501.
13. Khan A, Meyers JE, Yavorek S, et al. Comparing next-generation robotic technology with 3-dimensional computed tomography navigation technology for the insertion of posterior pedicle screws. World Neurosurg 2019;123:e474–81.
14. Zygourakis CC, Ahmed AK, Kalb S, et al. Technique: open lumbar decompression and fusion with the Excelsius GPS robot. Neurosurg Focus 2018;45(VideoSuppl1):V6.
15. Overley SC, Cho SK, Mehta AI, et al. Navigation and robotics in spinal surgery: where are we now? Neurosurgery 2017;80(3S):S86–99.

Minimally Invasive Advances in Deformity

David J. Mazur-Hart, MD, MS, Khoi D. Than, MD*

KEYWORDS

- Spinal deformity • MIS • Spinopelvic parameters • Osteotomy • Advances • Fusion • TLIF • LLIF

KEY POINTS

- Spinal deformity is a major cause of pain and disability in adults.
- Deformity correction using spinopelvic parameters is proven to decrease pain and disability, but these operations carry a high rate of morbidity and mortality.
- Minimally invasive approaches to deformity correction decrease operative morbidity without increasing health care spending.
- Continued technological advancements are increasing the number of approaches available to the minimally invasive spine surgeon while improving patient outcomes.

INTRODUCTION

Adult spinal deformity is a major contributor to pain and disability in the modern world. As the population continues to grow with increasing life expectancy, so does the burden of disease and disability. Not only are people living longer but they are healthier with greater expectations of function and activity. This demand to maintain performance status throughout adulthood and beyond retirement increases the demand to stay free of pain and disability. Surgical intervention for adult spinal deformity can both relieve pain and improve disability.

Spinal deformity is defined as having an abnormal curvature outside the accepted values of normal limits, which will be elucidated in later sections. Scoliosis is one well-defined form of spinal deformity in which the spine has a curvature greater than 10° in the coronal plane.[1] Scoliosis has numerous etiologies that vary based on patient demographics. The main etiologies include idiopathic, neuromuscular, syndromic, congenital, and degenerative.[2] This discussion primarily focuses on adult populations of spinal deformity. Adult scoliosis is defined as a curvature greater than 10° in a patient older than 18 years, although treatment is generally warranted for more severe cases. This form of deformity is primarily associated with degenerative etiologies, as the other listed etiologies are observed primarily in pediatric populations. These degenerative changes include spinal stenosis, spondylolisthesis, rotational subluxation, hyperlordosis, and rigidity.[3] Accelerated degeneration may come from asymmetric disk/facet degeneration or osteoporotic insufficiency fractures.

Previously, management of adult spinal deformity has included nonoperative interventions due to risks related to age, poor bone quality, and lack of adequate instrumentation/approaches. Patients wishing to remain active longer have pushed development of medical and surgical interventions to relieve pain and disability in this patient population. In this article, we discuss minimally invasive surgery (MIS) of the spine focusing on advancements in deformity correction.

EPIDEMIOLOGY

Adult degenerative scoliosis is a growing problem. As people live longer, there is cumulative burden of

---

Disclosures: Dr D.J. Mazur-Hart has nothing to disclosure. Dr K.D. Than is a consultant for Bioventus.
Department of Neurological Surgery, Oregon Health & Science University, Center for Health & Healing, CH8N, 3303 Southwest Bond Avenue, Portland, OR 97239, USA
* Corresponding author.
E-mail address: khoi.than@duke.edu

Neurosurg Clin N Am 31 (2020) 111–120
https://doi.org/10.1016/j.nec.2019.08.013

arthritic and degenerative changes. The total estimated US population is 327 million people (https://www.census.gov). Incidence and prevalence of adult spinal deformity have been difficult to establish due to the wide range of terminology used to describe degenerative changes of the spine. One study found prevalence of chronic low back pain to be 13.1% of US adults aged 20 to 69 years.[4] This group of people with chronic low back pain are heavy consumers of health care resources, with 23.8% having 10 or more different health care visits in the past year of the study compared with 10.4% of people without chronic low back pain. Persons 65 years and older represent roughly 15.6% of the population, or roughly 51 million people. Approximately, 68% of people older than 60 years have some degree of spinal deformity.[5] The reported incidence of spinal deformity is 37% of people aged 50 to 84 years.[6] The US population is not only growing, but life expectancy is estimated to continue to extend, which will increase the number of known spinal problems and create new areas of challenges to be solved.

SPINAL DEFORMITY PARAMETERS

Previous surgical interventions have focused on large, open, long-segment fusions to prevent worsening of the scoliotic deformity and to correct as much coronal deformity as possible without deficit (**Fig. 1**). These cases were primarily focused on younger patient populations with idiopathic scoliosis or progressive deformity from neuromuscular, syndromic, or congenital etiologies. As adult degenerative deformity has become more prevalent, interventions have focused on evidence-based improvements. Some of these goals of intervention have focused on spinopelvic parameters.

Spinopelvic parameters are measurements that identify the relationship of the spine to the pelvis. The pelvis has been identified as critically important to understanding spinal alignment. Abnormalities in this relationship can lead to cosmetic and symptomatic complaints. With corrected parameters, patients have improved pain and disability scores as well as quality of life. The most important spinopelvic parameters include sagittal vertical axis, pelvic tilt, pelvic incidence, and lumbar lordosis.

Sagittal vertical axis is the offset between a sagittal plumb line from the mid C7 vertebral body and a perpendicular line from the most posterosuperior corner of the sacrum (**Fig. 2**).[7] The ideal value is less than 5 cm, although normative values increase with age. Pelvic tilt is the angle between the line connecting the midpoint of the

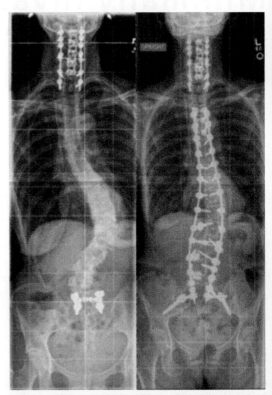

Fig. 1. Preoperative (*left*) and postoperative (*right*) standing AP films showing prior L5-S1 posterior instrumented fusion (PIF) with severe thoracolumbar scoliosis corrected by T5-ilium PIF, T4-T7 vertebroplasties, L4-L5 laminectomy, re-do L5-S1 laminectomy, L3-5 TLIF, and T12-L4 grade 1 osteotomies.

sacral endplate to the midpoint of the bicoxo-femoral axis and a vertical reference line (**Fig. 3**).[8] The ideal value is less than 20°, whereas higher values suggest pelvic retroversion to compensate for sagittal imbalance. Pelvic incidence is the angle between a line drawn perpendicular to the sacral end plate at its midpoint to a line drawn from the sacral end plate midpoint to the midpoint of the bicoxo-femoral axis (see **Fig. 3**).[9] This is a fixed number that does not change with intervention. Pelvic incidence helps to identify the ideal lumbar lordosis, which is a value that may change with intervention. Lumbar lordosis is the sagittal Cobb angle between the superior endplate of L1 and the sacral end plate (see **Fig. 2**).[10] Normal values range from roughly 40 to 60°. The goal value of lumbar lordosis is to be within 9° of the pelvic incidence. Sacral slope is the angle between the sacral end plate and a horizontal reference line (see **Fig. 3**).[11] Pelvic incidence is equal to the pelvic tilt summed with the sacral slope.[12]

With the exception of pelvic incidence, these parameters are able to be altered with deformity

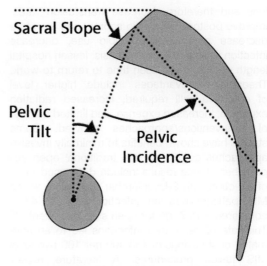

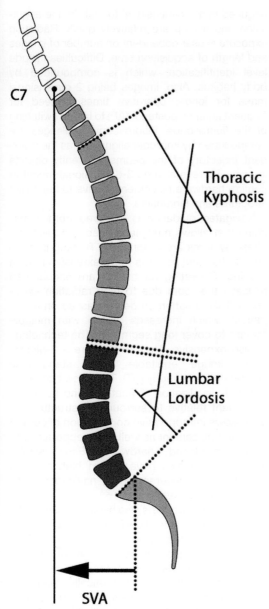

Fig. 2. Demonstrating parameters of sagittal vertical axis (SVA) and lumbar lordosis. Thoracic kyphosis also is demonstrated but not mentioned in this article. (*From* Klineberg E, Schwab F, Smith JS, et al. Sagittal spinal pelvic alignment. Neurosurg Clin N Am. 2013;24(2):158; with permission.)

Fig. 3. Demonstrating spinopelvic parameters of pelvic tilt, pelvic incidence, and sacral slope. (*From* Klineberg E, Schwab F, Smith JS, et al. Sagittal spinal pelvic alignment. Neurosurg Clin N Am. 2013;24(2):159; with permission.)

spinal cord deficit, nerve root deficit, vascular injury, visceral injury, instrumentation failure, junctional failure, deep wound infection, myocardial infarction, and neurologic deficit. Minor complications often include excessive blood loss, superficial infection, and cerebrospinal fluid leak.

Elderly individuals historically have had prohibitively high complication rates for any operative intervention, let alone spinal deformity correction. Some groups have found complication rates as high as 80%.[15] On the other hand, these patients show the greatest improvements in pain and disability following spinal deformity correction.[15]

MINIMALLY INVASIVE SURGERY APPLIED TO SPINAL DEFORMITY

Due to the high proportion of morbidity and increasingly frail populations indicated for adult spinal deformity correction, some surgeons have turned to minimally invasive approaches in the hopes of decreasing the perioperative morbidity and mortality rates from these procedures. MIS approaches are defined as those that minimize tissue disruption. MIS techniques should be able to achieve the same objectives as open techniques, which include adequate decompression, appropriately placed hardware, osseous fusion, and return of normal anatomic alignment. They also should be as safe as or safer than open approaches.

Theoretically, the advantages of less tissue disruption would decrease intraoperative blood

correction surgery. The potential problem with large, open deformity surgeries is the high rate of morbidity associated with them. Some studies have reported 30-day mortality rate of 2.4%.[13] Major complications have been recorded as roughly 10% to 15% in all adult populations with minor complication rates of 14% to 34%.[14] These major complications often include: cardiac arrest,

loss and therefore decrease transfusion rates, improve postoperative pain scores, and therefore decrease postoperative opioid use, decrease infection rates, improve cosmesis, lessen hospital length of stay, and lessen time to return to work. Theoretic disadvantages include higher level of operative skill required, increased radiation exposure, increased expense, and limited number of interventions/approaches allowed. Some studies have shown benefits to minimally invasive approaches compared with traditional open approaches. These results include decreased rates of infection with 2-level lumbar fusions, in which MIS patients had an infection rate of 4.6% compared with 7.0% for open surgery patients.[16] This rate of decreased infections led to an estimated cost savings of $38,400 per 100 two-level MIS fusion procedures. A literature review reported a surgical site infection rate of 0.6% for MIS transforaminal lumbar interbody fusion (TLIF) compared with 4.0% for open TLIF.[17] Another study found that patients receiving 2-level MIS fusion had a length of stay of 3.4 hospital days compared with 4.0 days for open 2-level fusion.[18] This correlated with another study by the same group that found MIS patients with single-level TLIF stayed 3.9 days and cost $70,159 compared with patients with open posterior lumbar interbody fusion, who stayed 4.8 days and cost $78,444.[19] Another group found their mean estimated blood loss (EBL) in posterior instrumented fusion cases with pedicle screw fixation to be 2.1 L with an average number of levels fused to be 4.7.[20] Another group reviewed their lateral lumbar interbody fusion (LLIF) procedures and found 8.4% of patients reached an EBL of 300 mL with an average number of levels fused to be 4.4.[21]

With rising health care costs, there will always be a continuous push for shorter procedure times and shorter length of hospital stays. Surgeons continue to pioneer new techniques and approaches while mastering established MIS techniques.

MINIMALLY INVASIVE PEDICLE SCREWS

One early adaptation of MIS techniques was screw placement in fusion surgery. Screws and rods can be placed percutaneously with minimal tissue disruption. With MIS placement, the entry point is unable to be visualized under direct visualization. Various techniques are used instead, including fluoroscopic as well as navigated guidance.

Fluoroscopic guidance is primarily the use of 1 or 2 C-arm machines using sequential or live fluoroscopic images.[2] This technique is well known with little additional training to staff. Images are acquired in a 2-dimensional format. Image acquisition and set up are relatively quick. Radiation exposure is user dependent on number of images and length of acquisition time. Difficulties include level identification, which is compounded by body habitus. Also, images being 2 dimensional make for longer operative times if need for frequent anterior-posterior (AP) to lateral switching of the fluoroscope. Fluoroscopy challenges are compounded by improper alignment, as the divergent trajectory of the beams inherently distorts images. There is also no 3-dimensional model to confirm hardware placement relative to important structures and landmarks.

Navigated guidance is acquired from a machine that allows multiplane image acquisition.[2] These systems are proprietary. Training is more substantial, and requires more extensive patient draping. Operating room staff are encouraged to leave the room due to high radiation exposures. This radiation burden is passed on to the patient, which increases greatly with multiple "spins" to cover long segments. The technology is also expensive. The benefits are a 3-dimensional image equitable to a stand-alone computed tomography (CT). This allows accurate detailed visualization of anatomy and hardware placement relative to surrounding structures. It also allows intraoperative confirmation of correct hardware placement as well as an opportunity to move misplaced hardware. Early single-institutional studies have shown high rates of pedicle screw accuracy using navigation while maintaining cost efficiency.[22,23]

Navigated guidance is also being combined with robotic technology to allow for further increases in accuracy of hardware placement. Navigational imaging can be uploaded to surgical robots. The robot is able to plan a trajectory and guide the screw placement, which theoretically lowers the amount of human error. Preliminary studies have shown noninferiority with equally high rates of pedicle screw accuracy to standard navigational placement.[24] Further analysis has trended toward superiority using robotic navigation.[25] The promise of robotic spine surgery is endless, including eventual assistance in performing dangerous osteotomy cuts.

All imaging modalities allow an estimation of coronal and sagittal correction, but neither allows visualization of correction given normal physiologic parameters. There are current software programs that allow preoperative calculation and manipulation of imaging to determine the amount of correction needed. This can be based on preoperative standing films, which simulates normal function versus prone intraoperative films. These programs have been found to have excellent predictive values of postoperative measurements.[26]

OSTEOTOMIES

A guiding principle of deformity surgery is correction of coronal and sagittal imbalance. As adult spinal deformity is classically from degenerative changes, the spine is usually characterized as rigid. This is opposed to adolescent scoliosis, which is usually a mobile deformity. The rigid spine must be mobilized to achieve proper alignment and balance. Mobilization can be caused by performing osteotomies. There are various grades of osteotomies classified by Schwab that allow for varying degrees of correction (**Table 1**).[27]

One of the perceived limitations of MIS is the lack of techniques to improve sagittal imbalance, which has previously been accomplished through open approaches. MIS techniques have been developed for both decompression and fixation/fusion. The following sections highlight advancements in MIS techniques for correcting sagittal imbalance.

Tubular Osteotomies (Grades 1 and 2)

Grade 1 and 2 osteotomies are collectively referred to as posterior column osteotomies. They focus on the removal of posterior elements with subsequent shortening of the posterior column. Grade 1 involves removal of the inferior facets. Grade 2 involves removal of both the superior and inferior articulating facets along with the ligamentum flavum and other posterior elements per surgeon preference (ie, spinous process, lamina). This is sometimes referred to as Ponte osteotomy, which was designed to shorten the posterior column to correct thoracic kyphosis, principally Scheuermann kyphosis. This is also sometimes referred to as Smith-Petersen osteotomy, which was described for correction of flat lumbar spine in ankylosing spondylitis. By removing all or part of the facet joint, the surgeon is able to compress across vertebral levels, which stretches the anterolateral ligament (ALL); accomplishing this requires a mobile disk space. Grade 1 and 2 osteotomies will generally allow for 5 to 10° of correction in the sagittal plane per level. These are technically safer than higher-grade osteotomies with less intraoperative blood loss, but require multiple levels of correction to achieve cumulative correction of sagittal vertical axis.

These techniques have classically been performed in open, multilevel fusion corrections. Minimally invasive techniques have been developed to achieve deformity correction with grade 1 and 2 osteotomies. This is primarily accomplished through an MIS TLIF. For degenerative pathology, this involves a unilateral approach with large dilators to remove the entire facet to access the disk space. This facetectomy can be performed on the contralateral side for correction of sagittal deformity. This MIS technique has been assisted by the innovation of expandable interbody grafts. They are passed through the dilators in the closed position. Once placed in the disk space, they are expanded to the appropriate height with strong loading pressure on both endplates. They also

Table 1
Grades of osteotomies and techniques

Osteotomy Grade	Nomenclature	Surgical Resection	Degrees of Correction
1	Partial facet joint osteotomy	Partial facet joint focused on the inferior facet	5
2	Smith-Petersen or Ponte (complete facet joint) osteotomy	Superior and inferior facets with ligamentum flavum and posterior elements	10
3	Pedicle subtraction osteotomy	Partial wedge resection through pedicle into vertebral body including posterior elements	20–30
4	More extensive pedicle subtraction osteotomy	Wider wedge resection including disk to endplate	30–40
5	Vertebral column resection	Complete removal of vertebral body including adjacent disks	40–60
6	Multiple vertebral column resections	Grade 5 and additional adjacent vertebral resection	60+

can be manufactured with hyperlordotic shapes to assist with the degree of correction required.

Mini-Open Pedicle Subtraction Osteotomy (Grade 3)

Grade 3 osteotomy is often referred to as a pedicle subtraction osteotomy (PSO). This extends the vertebral resection from just the posterior column to the anterior and middle columns. A wedge-shaped resection of bone is taken through the pedicle into the vertebral body. This allows for a larger amount of correction. A single-level PSO can achieve 30° of correction and asymmetric bony resection can correct coronal deformity. These 3-column osteotomies are associated with high degrees of morbidity. This stems from longer operation times with greater blood loss. The patient population is usually more deconditioned with greater deformity, and has had prior spine interventions. The neural elements are also exposed to a greater degree with greater instability of the spine until fixation.

Minimally invasive approaches to 3-column osteotomies would ideally decrease the amount of morbidity associated with these interventions. These approaches have been attempted in cadaveric models.[28] A mini-open approach has been developed and used in humans.[29] As described by the group, a long linear, midline incision is made with dissection to the fascia, as preferred over multiple stab incisions. For a grade 3 osteotomy in the lumbar spine, MIS TLIFs are performed at any number of levels below to promote bony fusion as well as further the degree of correction. At the level of the planned PSO, subperiosteal dissection is performed to the transverse processes with removal of the posterior elements. The exiting nerves above and below the targeted pedicle are identified and skeletonized to allow for protection. The pedicles are then drilled or taken by rongeurs to the dorsal vertebral body. Increasing sizes of curettes or osteotomes are used to remove a cone-shaped area of cancellous bone from the body. Sponges are used to dissect the lateral vertebral wall. Rongeurs are used to remove the lateral wall in wedge-shaped fashion similar to the cone of cancellous bone. This completes the osteotomy. The spine is stabilized with percutaneous pedicle screws at least 3 levels above and below the level of the osteotomy. This step is completed before final closure of the osteotomy. Once the rods are passed and secured with loosely tightened set screws, the posterior longitudinal ligament and posterior wall of the vertebral body are removed. This is accomplished by retracting the thecal sac medially from either side. Once the deformity is corrected, rod-to-rod connectors are attached where visible at the site of the PSO and the set screws are tightened. The group that described this approach has observed improvements in lumbar lordosis from 23.1 ± 15.9° to 48.6 ± 11.7° and sagittal vertical axis improvements from 102.4 ± 73.4 mm to 42.2 ± 39.9 mm[30]

LATERAL LUMBAR INTERBODY FUSION

Deformity correction surgery may also be accomplished through a lateral approach. These lateral approaches use small incisions with minimal tissue disruption. In comparison with posterior approaches, the posterior elements remain intact. They also should not interfere with peritoneal structures or the anterior longitudinal ligament like anterior approaches (ie, anterior lumbar interbody fusion [ALIF]). This lateral approach is termed LLIF, or minimally invasive lateral retroperitoneal transpsoas interbody fusion.

Lateral approaches have been developed because they allow for wide discectomy from endplate to endplate, which allows for the placement of large interbody grafts. Lateral approaches also allow for bilateral disruption of the annulus fibrosus, which facilitates coronal deformity correction. These large grafts theoretically allow for larger amounts of indirect neural decompression, greater deformity correction, improved fusion rates, and lower rates of subsidence. Studies have found similarly high rates of fusion; increased area of ipsilateral and contralateral neural foramen; and lower rates of subsidence and disk height loss with MIS LLIF compared with MIS TLIF.[31] These grafts can be stand-alone or can be combined with fixation. In adults, fixation devices are able to be placed laterally, but also can be fixated from subsequent posterior approaches with percutaneous pedicle screws and rods (**Fig. 4**). This allows for greater stability and allows for greater amounts of deformity correction. Single-level LLIF cages can correct roughly 5° in the sagittal plane per level compared with 2° corrected by TLIF.[32] Another review article of ALIF versus extreme lateral interbody fusion (XLIF) at L4-L5 found roughly 3° of correction by XLIF.[33]

The surgeon must be selective in choosing patients who would most benefit from a lateral approach. First, not all patients are candidates based on their own anatomy. A high-riding iliac crest may prohibit safe trajectory to the target levels. Another anatomic consideration is the lumbar plexus as it traverses the psoas muscle, but with the help of neuromonitoring, the risk of injury can be minimized.[34] Most neurologic issues will occur at the L4-L5 level.

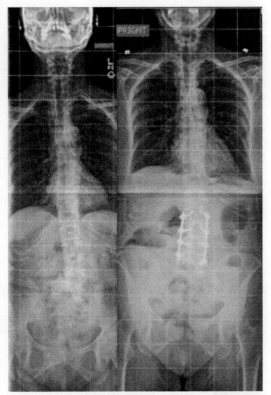

Fig. 4. Preoperative (*left*) and postoperative (*right*) standing AP films showing correction of scoliotic deformity with L2-L5 MIS LLIF and L2-L5 MIS PIF.

The approach is ideally from the side of the concavity to allow access to the maximum number of levels via the smallest incision, but this is debatable.[2,35] The patient is placed in the lateral position with the optimal side up. The legs are flexed to decrease tension on the iliopsoas muscle and nerves of the lumbosacral plexus. Rolls can be placed beneath the axilla and iliac crest. The patient is then taped securely to the table before breaking the table to open the disk spaces and increase the distance from the iliac crest to the lowest rib. Skin and fascia are sharply incised to access the targeted levels. Blunt dissection is carried in the retroperitoneal space until the psoas muscle is palpated. Sequential dilators are used with triggered electromyography in an attempt to avoid lumbar nerves and prevent injury. The retractor system is opened to allow for diskectomy and endplate preparation followed by placement of the interbody graft. It is imperative to maintain instruments as vertical as possible to limit injury to lumbar nerves posteriorly or vessels in the abdominal compartment anteriorly.

ANTERIOR COLUMN RELEASE

Another approach to lengthen the anterior column is to combine an MIS LLIF with the additional step of resecting the anterior longitudinal ligament, which has been termed anterior column release (ACR). One group found they were able to achieve 10 to 15° of correction per level in the sagittal plane with ALL release.[36] When combined with a posterior column osteotomy, even more correction can be accomplished (**Fig. 5**).

This MIS approach is taken through a lateral retroperitoneal or retropleural approach. Similar risks apply. First, the patient may experience a

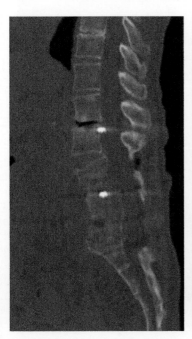
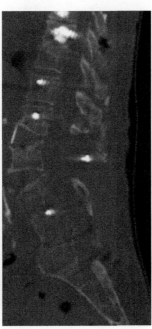

Fig. 5. Preoperative (*left*) and postoperative (*right*) CT lumbar spine without showing prior L2-S1 PIF with proximal junction kyphosis deformity corrected by L1-L3 LLIF, L1-L2 ACR, T10-ilium PIF, T9-10 vertebroplasties, L1-3 laminectomies, and L1-3 SPO.

nerve injury.[2] The lumbar plexus runs in and around the psoas muscle. Some of these at-risk nerves include the iliohypogastric, ilioinguinal, genitofemoral, and lateral femoral cutaneous nerves as they course across frequently accessed levels of L2-L4. Nerve injury also may occur to the sympathetic plexus, especially with the more extensive approach required for ACR. The genito-femoral and sympathetic plexus are difficult to monitor, as they do not have muscles to monitor reliably. Finally, vascular injury to the aorta or infe-rior vena cava may be catastrophic. Groups that perform this dissection recommend the ALL be sectioned with sharp dissection as opposed to electrocautery to prevent thermal injury to the nearby sensitive structures.

The procedure includes positioning the patient in the lateral decubitus position.[2] The retroperito-neal space is entered, followed by serial dilators into the psoas muscle aiming for the middle and posterior third of the disk space using electro-physiological monitoring to minimize risk of lumbar nerve plexus injury. This is followed by placement of a retractor secured to the table with shim blades

into the disk space. An annulotomy and diskec-tomy is performed. A curved custom retractor is then gently passed along the anterior edge of the ALL. This is placed between the large vessels and sympathetic chain ventrally and the disk space dorsally. A disk blade and intradiscal dis-tractor is used to section the ALL. Full division is confirmed when the endplates are easily mobilized and the ventral disk space has a "fish-mouth" opening. Then, a large hyperlordotic cage is placed depending on the degree of correction needed based on preoperative imaging. The inter-body is anchored into place with screws to avoid the risk of ventral migration of the interbody device into the peritoneal space.

LATERAL CORPECTOMY

Further correction may be obtained from a lateral approach with increasing grades of osteotomies, that is, grades 5 and 6. Because of the increasing amounts of instability with higher grades, they need to be combined with internal fixation, either from the same lateral approach or an additional

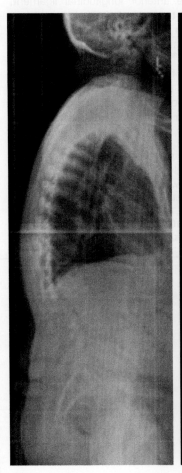
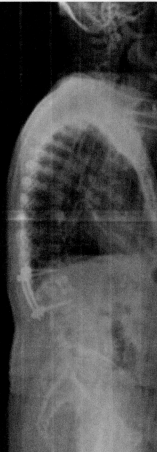

Fig. 6. Preoperative (*left*) and postop-erative (*right*) standing lateral radio-graphs showing L1 compression fracture with focal kyphosis corrected by L1 MIS lateral corpectomy and T12-L2 MIS PIF. The patient's focal kyphotic deformity improved from 32 to 19°.

posterior approach (**Fig. 6**). The patient is positioned laterally in similar steps as LLIF or ACR described previously, with a similar surgical approach. The target vertebral body is placed above the articulating point of the operating table and the retractor is targeted at the vertebral body.[37] If a rib is encountered, it may be dissected and removed. The discectomies are performed above and below followed by endplate preparation. This is followed by the corpectomy. The thecal sac is palpated to confirm adequate decompression. The cage may be chosen in a variety of forms including distractible cages for correction of deformity. If performing lateral fixation, this is performed after cage placement. If performing posterior fixation, the patient is positioned prone and performed either by an open or MIS approach.

SUMMARY

Adult spinal deformity is a growing problem in that it causes pain, disability, and exorbitant health care spending. Deformity surgery has been proven to decrease both pain and disability. Through technological advancements, minimally invasive approaches are being designed, which have been shown to decrease complications without increasing health care costs. These approaches have allowed patients in demographics considered prohibitive surgical candidates to undergo surgery and have excellent outcomes. Further research into techniques, technology, and patient outcomes remains important to developing spine surgery further and to increasing available surgical options.

REFERENCES

1. Silva FE, Lenke LG. Adult degenerative scoliosis: evaluation and management. Neurosurg Focus 2010;28(3):E1.
2. Wang MY, Lu Y, Anderson D, et al, editors. Minimally invasive spinal deformity surgery; an evolution of modern techniques. Vienna (Austria): Springer; 2014.
3. Lowe T, Berven SH, Schwab FJ, et al. The SRS classification for adult spinal deformity. Spine (Phila Pa 1976) 2006;31(Suppl):S119–25.
4. Shmagel A, Foley R, Ibrahim H. Epidemiology of chronic low back pain in US adults: data from the 2009-2010 National Health and Nutrition Examination Survey. Arthritis Care Res (Hoboken) 2016; 68(11):1688–94.
5. Schwab F, Dubey A, Gamez L, et al. Adult scoliosis: prevalence, SF-36, and nutritional parameters in an elderly volunteer population. Spine (Phila Pa 1976) 2005;30(9):1082–5.
6. Kobayashi T, Atsuta Y, Takemitsu M, et al. A prospective study of De Novo scoliosis in a community based cohort. Spine (Phila Pa 1976) 2006; 31(2):178–82.
7. Kuntz C, Levin LS, Ondra SL, et al. Neutral upright sagittal spinal alignment from the occiput to the pelvis in asymptomatic adults: a review and resynthesis of the literature. J Neurosurg Spine 2007; 6(2):104–12.
8. Lafage V, Schwab F, Patel A, et al. Pelvic tilt and truncal inclination. Spine (Phila Pa 1976) 2009; 34(17):E599–606.
9. Vialle R, Levassor N, Rillardon L, et al. Radiographic analysis of the sagittal alignment and balance of the spine in asymptomatic subjects. J Bone Joint Surg Am 2005;87(2):260–7.
10. Bernhardt M, Bridwell KH. Segmental analysis of the sagittal plane alignment of the normal thoracic and lumbar spines and thoracolumbar junction. Spine (Phila Pa 1976) 1989;14(7):717–21.
11. Berthonnaud E, Dimnet JS, Roussouly P, et al. Analysis of the sagittal balance of the spine and pelvis using shape and orientation parameters. J Spinal Disord Tech 2005;18(1):40–7.
12. Lafage V, Bharucha NJ, Schwab F, et al. Multicenter validation of a formula predicting postoperative spinopelvic alignment. J Neurosurg Spine 2012;16(1): 15–21.
13. Pateder DB, Gonzales RA, Kebaish KM, et al. Short-term mortality and its association with independent risk factors in adult spinal deformity surgery. Spine (Phila Pa 1976) 2008;33(11):1224–8.
14. Smith JS, Sansur CA, Donaldson WF, et al. Short-term morbidity and mortality associated with correction of thoracolumbar fixed sagittal plane deformity. Spine (Phila Pa 1976) 2011;36(12): 958–64.
15. Smith JS, Shaffrey CI, Glassman SD, et al. Risk-benefit assessment of surgery for adult scoliosis. Spine (Phila Pa 1976) 2011;36(10):817–24.
16. McGirt MJ, Parker SL, Lerner J, et al. Comparative analysis of perioperative surgical site infection after minimally invasive versus open posterior/transforaminal lumbar interbody fusion: analysis of hospital billing and discharge data from 5170 patients. J Neurosurg Spine 2011;14(6):771–8.
17. Parker SL, Adogwa O, Witham TF, et al. Post-operative infection after minimally invasive versus open transforaminal lumbar interbody fusion (TLIF): literature review and cost analysis. Minim Invasive Neurosurg 2011;54(01):33–7.
18. Wang MY, Lerner J, Lesko J, et al. Acute hospital costs after minimally invasive versus open lumbar interbody fusion. J Spinal Disord Tech 2012;25(6): 324–8.
19. Wang MY, Cummock MD, Yu Y, et al. An analysis of the differences in the acute hospitalization charges

following minimally invasive versus open posterior lumbar interbody fusion. J Neurosurg Spine 2010; 12(6):694–9.

20. Cho K-J, Suk S-I, Park S-R, et al. Complications in posterior fusion and instrumentation for degenerative lumbar scoliosis. Spine (Phila Pa 1976) 2007; 32(20):2232–7.

21. Phillips FM, Isaacs RE, Rodgers WB, et al. Adult degenerative scoliosis treated with XLIF. Spine (Phila Pa 1976) 2013;38(21):1853–61.

22. Luther N, Iorgulescu JB, Geannette C, et al. Comparison of navigated versus non-navigated pedicle screw placement in 260 patients and 1434 screws. J Spinal Disord Tech 2015;28(5): E298–303.

23. Shin BJ, James AR, Njoku IU, et al. Pedicle screw navigation: a systematic review and meta-analysis of perforation risk for computer-navigated versus freehand insertion. J Neurosurg Spine 2012;17(2): 113–22.

24. Kantelhardt SR, Martinez R, Baerwinkel S, et al. Perioperative course and accuracy of screw positioning in conventional, open robotic-guided and percutaneous robotic-guided, pedicle screw placement. Eur Spine J 2011;20(6):860–8.

25. Fan Y, Du JP, Liu JJ, et al. Accuracy of pedicle screw placement comparing robot-assisted technology and the free-hand with fluoroscopy-guided method in spine surgery. Medicine 2018;97(22):e10970.

26. Gupta M, Henry JK, Schwab F, et al. Dedicated spine measurement software quantifies key spinopelvic parameters more reliably than traditional picture archiving and communication systems tools. Spine (Phila Pa 1976) 2016;41(1):E22–7.

27. Schwab F, Blondel B, Chay E, et al. The comprehensive anatomical spinal osteotomy classification. Neurosurgery 2013;74(1):112–20.

28. Voyadzis J-M, Gala VC, O'Toole JE, et al. Minimally invasive posterior osteotomies. Neurosurgery 2008; 63(suppl_3):A204–10.

29. Wang MY, Madhavan K. Mini-open pedicle subtraction osteotomy: surgical technique. World Neurosurg 2014;81(5–6):843.e11-4.

30. Wang MY, Bordon G. Mini-open pedicle subtraction osteotomy as a treatment for severe adult spinal deformities: case series with initial clinical and radiographic outcomes. J Neurosurg Spine 2016;24(5): 769–76.

31. Isaacs RE, Sembrano J, Tohmeh AG. Two-year comparative outcomes of MIS lateral and MIS transforaminal interbody fusion in the treatment of degenerative spondylolisthesis: Part II: radiographic findings. Spine (Phila Pa 1976) 2016; 41(Suppl 8):S133–44.

32. Saadeh YS, Joseph JR, Smith BW, et al. Comparison of segmental lordosis and global spinopelvic alignment after single-level lateral lumbar interbody fusion or transforaminal lumbar interbody fusion. World Neurosurg 2019;126. e1374-8.

33. Winder MJ, Gambhir S. Comparison of ALIF vs. XLIF for L4/5 interbody fusion: pros, cons, and literature review. J Spine Surg 2016;2(1):2–8.

34. Uribe JS, Vale FL, Dakwar E. Electromyographic monitoring and its anatomical implications in minimally invasive spine surgery. Spine (Phila Pa 1976) 2010;35(Supplement):S368–74.

35. Baaj A, Mummaneni P, Uribe J, et al, editors. Handbook of spine surgery. New York, NY: Georg Thieme Verlag; 2016.

36. Deukmedjian AR, Dakwar E, Ahmadian A, et al. Early outcomes of minimally invasive anterior longitudinal ligament release for correction of sagittal imbalance in patients with adult spinal deformity. ScientificWorldJournal 2012; 2012:1–7.

37. Adkins DE, Sandhu FA, Voyadzis J-M. Minimally invasive lateral approach to the thoracolumbar junction for corpectomy. J Clin Neurosci 2013;20(9): 1289–94.

Robotic Tissue Manipulation and Resection in Spine Surgery

S. Joy Trybula, PharmD, MD, Daniel E. Oyon, MD, Jean-Paul Wolinsky, MD*

KEYWORDS

- Robotic • Spine • Neurosurgery • Surgical robot • Spinal tumor

KEY POINTS

- Image and navigation guidance has become increasingly used in neurosurgery and has paved the way for the introduction of surgical robots to the field.
- Navigation guidance systems are with increased accuracy in transpedicular screw placement; image guidance with an endoscope has been described for the resection of cervical, thoracic, and lumbar spine pathology.
- The US Food and Drug Administration approved 3 robotic systems for spine surgery, all of which provide the advantages of minimally invasive surgery.
- Although data for robotic-assisted resection of soft tissue spinal pathology are lacking, the da Vinci Surgical System has an increasing number of case reports and series supporting its safety and efficacy in spine surgery.
- The development of robotic tools for bone dissection would prove invaluable toward the use of robotic systems for spine surgery.

INTRODUCTION

Neurosurgery is a unique field that demands precisely applied force to penetrate dense osseous structures while carefully protecting delicate neurovascular structures within and surrounding the spinal cord and brain. Spine surgery in particular continues to be a physically demanding subspecialty that requires strenuous, repetitive tasks to correct spinal pathology. Over the past several decades, the introduction of image and navigation guidance systems in combination with surgical robotic assistants has raised interest in improving current standards of technique and accuracy in neurosurgery. As the use of intraoperative navigation in spine gained popularity for its accurate and safe placement of pedicle screws,[1–4] navigation guidance also came to be applied with increased frequency for the treatment of spinal tumors.

Arand and colleagues[5] (2002) became the first to use navigation for the decompression and pedicle screw placement of metastatic thoracic spinal tumors through a pair-point matching technique used to superimpose the preoperative computed tomography dataset onto a dynamic intraoperative reference base. Vougioukas and colleagues[6] (2003) used an occlusal splint registration system for the transoral resection of 3 craniocervical chordomas, as well as for medullary decompression in a case of rheumatoid atlantoaxial subluxation. Smitherman and colleagues[7]

Disclosure: The authors have nothing to disclose.
Department of Neurological Surgery, Northwestern University, Feinberg School of Medicine, 676 North St. Clair Street, Suite 2210, Chicago, IL 60611-2292, USA
* Corresponding author. Department of Neurosurgery, Northwestern University, Feinberg School of Medicine, 676 North St. Clair Street, Suite 2210, Chicago, IL 60611-2292.
E-mail addresses: jean-paul.wolinsky@northwestern.edu; jpw@nm.org

neurosurgery.theclinics.com

(2010) were among the first to describe the use of navigation guidance for creating osteotomies during the en bloc resection of a malignant giant cell tumor, and Fujibayashi and colleagues[8] (2010) used similar methods for en bloc resection of various solitary malignant spinal tumors, as well as a case of kyphotic deformity of ankylosing spondylitis. Additionally, a number of studies have published promising results using a variety of navigation modalities (frameless stereotaxis with gamma-probe guidance, fluoroscopy, Siremobil Iso-C 3D arm, or O-arm) and computer systems (Medtronic's StealthStation [Medtronic, Dublin, Ireland] or BrainLAB's VectorVision [Vector Laboratories, Burlingame, CA]) for the high-speed drill excision of osteoid osteomas and osteoblastomas.[9–14] Bandiera and colleagues[15] (2013) used both Medtronic and BrainLAB systems to successfully resect a combination of primary and metastatic spinal tumors among seven patients without complications. Since then, multiple surgeons have begun using coregistration of preoperative MRI with intraoperative computed tomography imaging to more accurately define tumor borders and displaced normal soft tissue anatomy, thereby facilitating safe tumor resection and instrumentation.[16,17] In one of the largest studies to date, Nasser and colleagues[18] (2016) demonstrated the efficacy of the StealthStation with O-arm integration on a multicenter analysis of 50 patients with both primary and metastatic spinal column tumors, with no intraoperative complications, and one postoperative death from pulmonary embolism in the metastatic group.

Image guidance with the use of an endoscope for the resection of cervical, thoracic, and lumbosacral spine pathology has also gained much support over the years. Wolinsky and colleagues[19] (2007) and McGirt and colleagues[20] (2008) reported successful odontoidectomy using transcervical endoscopy in a series of patients with basilar invagination. BrainLAB navigation has also been used in conjunction with an endoscope for the intralesional resection of a cervical chordoma, as well as for guidance for osteotomies in en bloc resection of sacral chordomas.[21,22] Many tumors of the thoracic spine such as nerve sheath tumors, osteoid osteomas, and schwannomas have also been successfully treated via combined video-assisted thoracoscopy and Stealth navigation.[23–25] Last, despite the rarity of spinal tumors with sacral or pelvic involvement, endoscopy for such tumors have been particularly well-described in the literature, with a plethora of case reports reporting uncomplicated resection of benign presacral or retroperitoneal masses such as nerve sheath tumors and ganglioneuromas.[26–31] Overall, these various modalities and applications of image guidance have paved the way for the introduction of robotics into neurosurgical practice.

Nathoo and colleagues[32] (2005) classified robotic assistance into 3 broad categories based on how the surgeon interacts with them: (1) supervisory-controlled systems, in which the surgeon plans the operation and the machine carries out the programmed, predetermined actions with surgeon supervision, (2) telesurgical systems (such as the da Vinci Surgical System, Intuitive Surgical, Sunnyvale, CA), in which the robot is under direct control of the surgeon from a remote command station during the operation and the surgeon's actions are executed faithfully by the robot in real time, and (3) shared control systems, a form of co-autonomy where the surgeon remains in control of the procedure and the robot provides steady-hand manipulation of surgical instruments. Currently, the majority of robots designed for use in spine surgery exercise shared control systems, with the exception of the da Vinci robot, which has been primarily used for tumor resection owing to superior 3-dimensional visualization, bimanual dissection with wristed instruments, and the ability to use a second assistant at the patient's side. We present a review of the currently available robotic assistants for navigation in spine surgery and present the currently available evidence for robotic use in spinal tissue manipulation and resection.

ROBOTIC ASSISTANCE IN SPINE TUMOR SURGERY

Since the advent of image, navigation, and endoscopic guidance for the treatment of spinal pathology, much emphasis has been placed on increasing the accuracy and safety of such procedures. Increasing the precision of dissection has long been a focal point in neurosurgery and, to this end, robotic technology has revealed itself to be an invaluable tool for the application of minimally invasive techniques and tissue-sparing surgery. As highlighted, there is a growing body of data regarding the safety and efficacy of robotic assistance in transpedicular screw placement and instrumentation, particularly with the use of Mazor's SpineAssist, Renaissance, and Mazor X robot systems (Mazor Robotics, Caesarea, Israel). The data for robotic soft tissue surgery in spine, however, is lacking. This is attributed to the relative rarity of spinal tumors compared with degenerative changes of the spine, as well as to the extensive subspecialization required to become proficient in neurosurgical robotics.

The most widely used surgical robot today is the da Vinci Surgical System (Intuitive Surgical). Originally approved by the US Food and Drug Administration in 2000 for general laparoscopic procedures, the da Vinci Surgical System was designed as a telesurgical instrument by which the surgeon operates the robot as an extension of his or her body from a remote booth, and has enjoyed widespread use in urologic and gynecologic procedures. In the spinal realm, the da Vinci robot has been used for anterior lumbar interbody fusion, with a number of case series demonstrating excellent safety profiles in avoiding neurologic, vascular, or ureteral injury during the procedure.[33–35] The data for da Vinci-assisted spine tumor resection, however, have also increased. **Table 1** lists all the relevant cases and case series depicted in the literature regarding the use of robotic assistance for the surgical resection of spine tumors, as well as a case of basilar invagination.[34–48] Of note, the majority of cases consisted of benign pathologies.

The first reported case of robotic-assisted spine surgery for tumor resection was conducted by Ruurda and colleagues[36] (2003), who used the da Vinci system via thoracoscopy for the gross total resection of a thoracic ancient schwannoma without complication. The da Vinci-assisted thoracoscopic approach for thoracic tumors has since been validated by multiple authors with no reported morbidity.[37,42,46] Complex intraspinal tumors with thoracic extension can also be treated with a combination of posterior freehand osseous decompression or tumor debulking followed by anterior excision of the thoracic component.[41] A case of retroperitoneal transdiaphragmatic robotic-assisted laparoscopy has even been described for the resection of a neurofibroma in the T12 to L1 paraspinal area abutting the hemidiaphragm and kidney.[38] Functionally, robotic assistance can be achieved within any body cavity that is accessible with an endoscope through minimally invasive incisions. As such, similar to the literature surrounding navigation guidance for laparoscopic resection of lumbosacral tumors, there is a growing body of case reports supporting robotic-assisted transperitoneal laparoscopy for tumors with pelvic involvement. In the case of benign lesions such as schwannomas, ganglioneuromas, and neurofibromas, da Vinci-assisted resection has demonstrated great efficacy in achieving gross total resection without morbidity.[40,45,47–49] Oh and colleagues[43] (2014) directly compared the efficacy of robotic-assisted resection of huge (diameter >10 cm) presacral masses with that of conventional open transperitoneal resection. Gross total resection

was achieved in all cases of benign tumors for both groups, but robotic-assisted resection was associated with shorter duration of surgery, markedly less bleeding, shorter hospitalization, and shorter recovery time.

Robotic assistance has seen occasional use for osseous resection as well. Bederman and colleagues[44] (2014) achieved an en bloc resection of a sacral osteosarcoma through a combined anteroposterior approach in which pilot holes were drilled across the planned iliac resection margin using navigation with Renaissance, with rigid tubes subsequently placed into the pilot holes and a series of osteotomes passed through the navigation-guided tubes to complete the osteotomy. A successful transoral robotic odontoidectomy has also been described for the treatment of basilar invagination using the da Vinci Surgical System; however, robotic assistance was used for soft tissue exposure and the drilling was performed freehand with a standard drill.[39] Although data exist to support the accuracy of robotic pedicle screw placement in the setting of malignancy,[50] robotic surgery for resection of bony tumors remains limited and poorly studied owing to the limitations imposed by a minimally invasive approach.

Advantages and Disadvantages of Robotic Spine Surgery

The application of robotic assistance toward definitive resection of soft tissue spine tumors affords the surgeon numerous distinct advantages over a conventional approach. Of the current commercially available robots, the endoscopically driven da Vinci Surgical System has been used most frequently for the excision of benign spinal pathology. First, the da Vinci offers all the advantages of minimally invasive surgery, including smaller incisions, decreased tissue trauma and bleeding, protection of normal neurovascular anatomy, decrease pain, and a shorter length of stay and functional recovery time. Equally important, the da Vinci provides enhanced visualization simply unrivaled by conventional or navigation-guided surgery. The 3-dimensional properties, illumination, and depth perception that the binocular endoscopic camera provides exquisite visualization of structures, which can be magnified into the 12× to 40× range.[38] This enhanced view facilitates accurate and safe dissection as well as easier coagulation of vessels, thereby decreasing the risk of iatrogenic injury to normal anatomy. Unlike a traditional endoscope, the da Vinci camera is controlled by the operating surgeon at the remote console with hands-free controls, elimination of

Table 1
Studies of spinal and paraspinal tumor or bony resection utilizing robotic assistance

Authors, Year	Study	Robotic Modality	n	Approach/Procedure	Pathology	Outcome
Ruurda et al,[36] 2003	Case report	da Vinci	1	Thoracoscopy	Thoracic "ancient" schwannoma	Gross total resection, no complications
Morgan et al,[37] 2003	Case series	da Vinci	2	Thoracoscopy	Neurofibroma, schwannoma	Gross total resection of both tumors, no complications
Moskowitz et al,[38] 2009	Case report	da Vinci	1	Retroperitoneal transdiaphragmatic laparoscopy	Thoracolumbar neurofibroma	Gross total resection, no complications
Lee et al,[39] 2010	Case report	da Vinci	1	Transoral robotic odontoidectomy	Basilar invagination	Full decompression of craniocervical junction, no complications
Yang et al,[40] 2011	Case report	da Vinci	1	Transperitoneal laparoscopy	Lumbar paraspinal schwannoma	Gross total resection, no complications
Perez-Cruet et al,[41] 2012	Case series	da Vinci	2	Combined posterior freehand and anterior robotic approach	Thoracic paraspinal schwannomas	Gross total resection of both tumors, no complications
Finley et al,[42] 2014	Case report	da Vinci	1	Thoracoscopy	Thoracic paraspinal schwannoma	Gross total resection, no complications
Oh et al,[43] 2014	Case series	da Vinci	5	Transperitoneal laparoscopy	Huge (diameter >10 cm) presacral tumors (3 schwannomas, 1 malignant neurofibroma, 1 transitional meningioma)	4 gross total resections and 1 near-total resection (malignant involvement of nerve root), 1 patient developed postoperative numbness and 1 developed neuropathic pain
Bederman et al,[44] 2014	Case report	Renaissance	1	Robotic-assisted osteotomies for en bloc sacrectomy	Sacral osteosarcoma	En bloc resection, no complications (post-sacrectomy bowel/bladder incontinence expected)

Palep et al,[45] 2015	Case report	da Vinci	1	Transperitoneal laparoscopy	Precoccygeal ganglioneuroma	Gross total resection, no complications
Pacchiarotti et al,[46] 2017	Case series	da Vinci	2	Thoracoscopy	Thoracic paravertebral schwannomas	Gross total resection of both tumors, no complications
Yin et al,[47] 2018	Case series	da Vinci	7	Transperitoneal laparoscopy; 2 cases followed by posterior freehand approach	Sacral/presacral tumors (5 schwannomas, 1 chordoma, 1 solitary fibroma)	5 gross total resections and 2 near-total resections (1 schwannoma, 1 chordoma), no complications
Jun et al,[48] 2018	Operative video, case report	da Vinci	1	Transperitoneal laparoscopy	Presacral schwannoma	Gross total resection, no complications
Garzon-Muvdi et al,[49] 2018	Case report	da Vinci	1	Transperitoneal laparoscopy	Presacral ganglioneuroma	Near-total resection (residual extension into S2 neural foramen), no complications
Petrov et al,[50] 2019	Case report	da Vinci	1	Transoral robotic exposure with freehand en bloc resection and instrumentation	Cervical chordoma	En bloc resection; pharyngeal wound dehiscence and infection, no permanent complications

untoward movement, and a wider field of view. This optimum field of view is particularly helpful when operating in narrow corridors such as the pelvis, even in the presence of a large mass.[49] Additionally, robotic surgery confers a unique and invaluable advantage in the reduction of human error. The surgeon's movements at the console are instantaneously translated to robotic arm movements with up to 1:5 motion scaling, allowing the user to make the finest of movements in a highly controlled fashion. The robot computer is also able to eliminate any hand tremor automatically and provides the surgeon with 540° of wrist action, granting enhanced control over the surgical field. The robotic arms themselves have 6 degrees of freedom for superior maneuverability at great depth in the surgical field, and the wristed dissectors permit the robotic arms to make acute-angled reaches around anatomic constraints. The primary surgeon at the console can also be assisted by a bedside surgeon who facilitates transfer of instruments and retraction through a manual-assistant port. Last, the surgeon's console provides optimal ergonomics in a seated working environment free of sterile draping, which can lead to improved comfort and reduced operative fatigue.

Despite its numerous advantages, da Vinci-assisted surgery is not without limitations. The most pertinent disadvantage to the applicability of spinal surgery is the lack of instruments for bone dissection. The 3 robotic arms are typically inserted through 3 separate trocar ports for access; however, there are currently no existing drill attachments for the robot arms capable of traversing minimally invasive ports. Thus, the da Vinci is not a viable modality for primary bone tumors, malignant tumors with osseous involvement, or metastatic spine tumors and is instead ideal for benign soft tissue masses. It is certainly possible to use the da Vinci system for safe soft tissue exposures in narrow, delicate anatomic areas such as the oropharynx followed by freehand resection, as described by Petrov and colleagues[51] (2019) for the transoral en bloc resection of a cervical chordoma. Another equipment-related disadvantage of da Vinci-assisted spine surgery is the lack of dedicated robot- arm tools for intraoperative nerve monitoring. Garzon-Muvdi and colleagues[49] (2018) circumvented this problem by using the bipolar forceps as the stimulating probe when coupled to a nerve stimulation system. Despite a relative lack of diversity in attachable instruments for the da Vinci robot arm, these studies show that adaptable techniques exist to incorporate robotic assistance for a variety of procedures. Moreover, research is being conducted toward the development of new instruments such as prototype burrs and rongeurs, which has the potential to permit neurosurgeons to perform da Vinci-assisted bone dissection or posterior approach procedures for spine patients.[52]

Other disadvantages of the da Vinci system include the lack of haptic feedback. Despite a lack of physical and sensory feedback from controlling the robot arms remotely, the superb 3-dimensional high definition afforded by the binocular endoscope has been shown to create the subjective perception of haptics among both novices and experienced robotic surgeons.[53] Last, the acquisition cost of the da Vinci machine remains quite high and thus requires a high-volume practice setting to justify the investment. Advanced subspecialty training in an academic environment is also required, although studies on da Vinci-assisted urologic procedures have demonstrated short learning curves for surgeons learning the technique.[54] Although the vast majority of the literature on robotic assistance for surgical spine tumor treatment surrounds the da Vinci robot, a small number of studies have demonstrated the use of Mazor robotics for pedicle screw placement to provide spinal stability in the setting of malignancy.[50,55,56] Further studies are needed to explore the possible applications of both da Vinci and Mazor-assisted spine surgery, particularly alongside the development of new surgical robotic arms and instruments for bone dissection.

SUMMARY

Robots have the potential to become an excellent resource for spine surgeons because of their potential for superior precision, improved visualization, and resistance to fatigue. These advantages have been applied to resection of sacral masses deep within the pelvis. Additionally, because neurosurgeons are interested in and capable of removing larger tumors, revising prior operative complications, and handling larger deformity cases with distorted anatomy, robots may become increasingly useful as a resource for complex or revision cases. Robotic use in spine surgery has impressively evolved since the 1990s, and with the continued trend of improving technology and imaging software, we may expect robots to play a larger role as experience accumulates and long-term cost effectiveness is proven.

The ideal robot would be capable of promoting adjustable autonomy, submillimeter accuracy, minimal invasiveness, low radiation doses, and ease of registration and image guidance. Obstacles to current implementation of robotics in spine surgery include a maximum of 3 operative spinal levels, existing evidence primarily for lumbar instrumentation placement, difficulty with cost effectiveness, and a learning curve of at least 30 cases to decrease radiation exposure and operative time.[57] As robotic assistance becomes increasingly used for the resection of benign spinal and paraspinal tumors, simultaneous development of robotic-compatible instruments for bone dissection could pave the way for a new era of robotic-assisted spine surgery. As demonstrated by an increasing number of case reports and series, the da Vinci robot confers clear advantages in tight operative corridors that human hands physically may not be able to reach or that require heightened physical stamina to expose the surgical field. In the included table of studies reporting the use of the Da Vinci robot for paraspinal tumor resection, the main commonality was the complexity of tumor location (ie, high cervical, upper to mid-thoracic, or presacral). These technically challenging locations present ideal opportunities to use a telesurgical robotic design that greatly decreases operator fatigue. Of course, there remain disadvantages to the da Vinci system; however, we expect that the next few decades will continue to produce more software and hardware advances that may make telesurgical robots more common in spine surgery. Patients and surgeons alike are increasingly interested in minimally invasive methods to reduce morbidity, cost, and operative time. The full acceptance and implementation of these tools are dependent on clinical evidence and literature that supports their value.

REFERENCES

1. Verma R, Krishan S, Haendlmayer K, et al. Functional outcome of computer-assisted spinal pedicle screw placement: a systematic review and meta-analysis of 23 studies including 5,992 pedicle screws. Eur Spine J 2010;19(3):370–5.
2. Shin BJ, James AR, Njoku IU, et al. Pedicle screw navigation: a systematic review and meta-analysis of perforation risk for computer-navigated versus freehand insertion. J Neurosurg Spine 2012;17(2): 113–22.
3. Gelalis ID, Paschos NK, Pakos EE, et al. Accuracy of pedicle screw placement: a systematic review of prospective in vivo studies comparing free hand, fluoroscopy guidance and navigation techniques. Eur Spine J 2012;21(2):247–55.
4. Aoude AA, Fortin M, Figueiredo R, et al. Methods to determine pedicle screw placement accuracy in spine surgery: a systematic review. Eur Spine J 2015;24(5):990–1004.
5. Arand M, Hartwig E, Kinzl L, et al. Spinal navigation in tumor surgery of the thoracic spine: first clinical results. Clin Orthop Relat Res 2002;399:211–8.
6. Vougioukas VI, Hubbe U, Schipper J, et al. Navigated transoral approach to the cranial base and the craniocervical junction: technical note. Neurosurgery 2003;52(1):247–50 [discussion: 251].
7. Smitherman SM, Tatsui CE, Rao G, et al. Image-guided multilevel vertebral osteotomies for en bloc resection of giant cell tumor of the thoracic spine: case report and description of operative technique. Eur Spine J 2010;19(6):1021–8.
8. Fujibayashi S, Neo M, Takemoto M, et al. Computer-assisted spinal osteotomy: a technical note and report of four cases. Spine (Phila Pa 1976) 2010; 35(18):E895–903.
9. Van Royen BJ, Baayen JC, Pijpers R, et al. Osteoid osteoma of the spine: a novel technique using combined computer-assisted and gamma probe-guided high-speed intralesional drill excision. Spine (Phila Pa 1976) 2005;30(3):369–73.
10. Moore T, McLain RF. Image-guided surgery in resection of benign cervicothoracic spinal tumors: a report of two cases. Spine J 2005;5(1):109–14.
11. Rajasekaran S, Kamath V, Shetty AP. Intraoperative Iso-C three-dimensional navigation in excision of spinal osteoid osteomas. Spine (Phila Pa 1976) 2008;33(1):E25–9.
12. Rajasekaran S, Kanna RM, Kamath V, et al. Computer navigation-guided excision of cervical osteoblastoma. Eur Spine J 2010;19(6):1046–7.
13. Nagashima H, Nishi T, Yamane K, et al. Case report: osteoid osteoma of the C2 pedicle: surgical technique using a navigation system. Clin Orthop Relat Res 2010;468(1):283–8.
14. Mori K, Neo M, Takemoto M, et al. Navigated pinpoint approach to osteoid osteoma adjacent to the facet joint of spine. Asian Spine J 2016;10(1): 158–63.
15. Bandiera S, Ghermandi R, Gasbarrini A, et al. Navigation-assisted surgery for tumors of the spine. Eur Spine J 2013;22(Suppl 6):S919–24.
16. D'Andrea K, Dreyer J, Fahim DK. Utility of preoperative magnetic resonance imaging coregistered with intraoperative computed tomographic scan for the resection of complex tumors of the spine. World Neurosurg 2015;84(6):1804–15.
17. Maduri R, Bobinski L, Duff JM. Image Merge Tailored Access Resection (IMTAR) of spinal intradural tumors. Technical report of 13 cases. World Neurosurg 2017;98:594–602.
18. Nasser R, Drazin D, Nakhla J, et al. Resection of spinal column tumors utilizing image-guided navigation: a multicenter analysis. Neurosurg Focus 2016; 41(2):E15.
19. Wolinsky JP, Sciubba DM, Suk I, et al. Endoscopic image-guided odontoidectomy for decompression

of basilar invagination via a standard anterior cervical approach. Technical note. J Neurosurg Spine 2007;6(2):184–91.

20. McGirt MJ, Attenello FJ, Sciubba DM, et al. Endoscopic transcervical odontoidectomy for pediatric basilar invagination and cranial settling. Report of 4 cases. J Neurosurg Pediatr 2008;1(4):337–42.

21. Hsu W, Kosztowski TA, Zaidi HA, et al. Image-guided, endoscopic, transcervical resection of cervical chordoma. J Neurosurg Spine 2010;12(4):431–5.

22. Dasenbrock HH, Clarke MJ, Bydon A, et al. En bloc resection of sacral chordomas aided by frameless stereotactic image guidance: a technical note. Neurosurgery 2012;70(1 Suppl Operative):82–7 [discussion: 87–8].

23. Ghostine S, Vaynman S, Schoeb JS, et al. Image-guided thoracoscopic resection of thoracic dumbbell nerve sheath tumors. Neurosurgery 2012;70(2):461–7 [discussion: 468].

24. Campos WK, Gasbarrini A, Boriani S. Case report: curetting osteoid osteoma of the spine using combined video-assisted thoracoscopic surgery and navigation. Clin Orthop Relat Res 2013;471(2):680–5.

25. Johnson JP, Drazin D, King WA, et al. Image-guided navigation and video-assisted thoracoscopic spine surgery: the second generation. Neurosurg Focus 2014;36(3):E8.

26. Kohler C, Kuhne-Heid R, Klemm P, et al. Resection of presacral ganglioneurofibroma by laparoscopy. Surg Endosc 2003;17(9):1499.

27. Konstantinidis K, Theodoropoulos GE, Sambalis G, et al. Laparoscopic resection of presacral schwannomas. Surg Laparosc Endosc Percutan Tech 2005;15(5):302–4.

28. Yang CC, Chen HC, Chen CM. Endoscopic resection of a presacral schwannoma. Case report. J Neurosurg Spine 2007;7(1):86–9.

29. Kang CM, Kim DH, Seok JY, et al. Laparoscopic resection of retroperitoneal benign schwannoma. J Laparoendosc Adv Surg Tech A 2008;18(3):411–6.

30. Champney MS, Ehteshami M, Scales FL. Laparoscopic resection of a presacral ganglioneuroma. Am Surg 2010;76(4):E1–2.

31. Gorgun M, Sezer TO, Kirdok O. Laparoscopic resection of retroperitoneal schwannoma near the inferior vena. Ann Vasc Surg 2010;24(4):551.e1-4.

32. Nathoo N, Çavuşoğlu MC, Vogelbaum MA, et al. Touch with robotics: neurosurgery for the future. Neurosurgery 2005;56(3):421–33.

33. Lee Z, Lee JY, Welch WC, et al. Technique and surgical outcomes of robot-assisted anterior lumbar interbody fusion. J Robot Surg 2013;7(2):177–85.

34. Lee JY, Bhowmick DA, Eun DD, et al. Minimally invasive, robot-assisted, anterior lumbar interbody fusion: a technical note. J Neurol Surg A Cent Eur Neurosurg 2013;74(4):258–61.

35. Beutler WJ, Peppelman WC Jr, DiMarco LA. The da Vinci robotic surgical assisted anterior lumbar interbody fusion: technical development and case report. Spine (Phila Pa 1976) 2013;38(4):356–63.

36. Ruurda JP, Hanlo PW, Hennipman A, et al. Robot-assisted thoracoscopic resection of a benign mediastinal neurogenic tumor: technical note. Neurosurgery 2003;52(2):462–4 [discussion: 464].

37. Morgan JA, Kohmoto T, Smith CR, et al. Endoscopic computer-enhanced mediastinal mass resection using robotic technology. Heart Surg Forum 2003;6(6):E164–6.

38. Moskowitz RM, Young JL, Box GN, et al. Retroperitoneal transdiaphragmatic robotic-assisted laparoscopic resection of a left thoracolumbar neurofibroma. JSLS 2009;13(1):64–8.

39. Lee JY, Lega B, Bhowmick D, et al. Da Vinci Robot-assisted transoral odontoidectomy for basilar invagination. ORL J Otorhinolaryngol Relat Spec 2010;72(2):91–5.

40. Yang MS, Kim KN, Yoon DH, et al. Robot-assisted resection of paraspinal Schwannoma. J Korean Med Sci 2011;26(1):150–3.

41. Perez-Cruet MJ, Welsh RJ, Hussain NS, et al. Use of the da Vinci minimally invasive robotic system for resection of a complicated paraspinal schwannoma with thoracic extension: case report. Neurosurgery 2012;71(1 Suppl Operative):209–14.

42. Finley D, Sherman JH, Avila E, et al. Thorascopic resection of an apical paraspinal schwannoma using the da Vinci surgical system. J Neurol Surg A Cent Eur Neurosurg 2014;75(1):58–63.

43. Oh JK, Yang MS, Yoon DH, et al. Robotic resection of huge presacral tumors: case series and comparison with an open resection. J Spinal Disord Tech 2014;27(4):E151–4.

44. Bederman SS, Lopez G, Ji T, et al. Robotic guidance for en bloc sacrectomy: a case report. Spine (Phila Pa 1976) 2014;39(23):E1398–401.

45. Palep JH, Mistry S, Kumar A, et al. Robotic excision of a pre-coccygeal nerve root tumor. J Minim Access Surg 2015;11(1):103–5.

46. Pacchiarotti G, Wang MY, Kolcun JPG, et al. Robotic paravertebral schwannoma resection at extreme locations of the thoracic cavity. Neurosurg Focus 2017;42(5):E17.

47. Yin J, Wu H, Tu J, et al. Robot-assisted sacral tumor resection: a preliminary study. BMC Musculoskelet Disord 2018;19(1):186.

48. Jun C, Sukumaran M, Wolinsky JP. Robot-assisted resection of pre-sacral schwannoma. Neurosurg Focus 2018;45(VideoSuppl1):V1.

49. Garzon-Muvdi T, Belzberg A, Allaf ME, et al. Intraoperative nerve monitoring in robotic-assisted resection of presacral ganglioneuroma: operative

technique. Oper Neurosurg (Hagerstown) 2019;
16(1):103–10.

50. Hu X, Scharschmidt TJ, Ohnmeiss DD, et al. Robotic
assisted surgeries for the treatment of spine tumors.
Int J Spine Surg 2015;9. https://doi.org/10.14444/
2001.

51. Petrov D, Spadola M, Berger C, et al. Novel approach
using ultrasonic bone curettage and transoral robotic
surgery for en bloc resection of cervical spine chordoma: case report. J Neurosurg Spine 2019;1–6.
https://doi.org/10.3171/2018.11.spine181162.

52. Ponnusamy K, Chewning S, Mohr C. Robotic approaches to the posterior spine. Spine (Phila Pa
1976) 2009;34(19):2104–9.

53. Hagen ME, Meehan JJ, Inan I, et al. Visual clues act
as a substitute for haptic feedback in robotic surgery. Surg Endosc 2008;22(6):1505–8.

54. Artibani W, Fracalanza S, Cavalleri S, et al. Learning
curve and preliminary experience with da Vinci-
assisted laparoscopic radical prostatectomy. Urol
Int 2008;80(3):237–44.

55. Booher G, Vardiman A. Navigated robotic assisted
thoracic pedicle screw placement for metastatic
renal cell carcinoma. Neurosurg Focus 2018;
45(VideoSuppl1):V5.

56. Parker SL, McGirt MJ, Farber SH, et al. Accuracy
of free-hand pedicle screws in the thoracic and
lumbar spine: analysis of 6816 consecutive
screws. Neurosurgery 2011;68(1):170–8 [discus-
sion: 178].

57. Hu X, Lieberman IH. What is the learning curve for
robotic-assisted pedicle screw placement in spine
surgery? Clin Orthop Relat Res 2014;472(6):
1839–44.

Cell and Gene Therapy for Spine Regeneration
Mammalian Protein Production Platforms for Overproduction of Therapeutic Proteins and Growth Factors

Ali Mobasheri, BSc, ARCS, MSc, DPhil (Oxon)[a,b,c,d,*],
Stephen M. Richardson, BSc, PhD[e]

KEYWORDS

- Low back pain (LBP) • Spine degeneration • Cell therapy • Gene therapy
- Mammalian protein production platforms • Protein packaging cell lines • Growth factors
- Transforming growth factor-β (TGF-β) • GDF6

KEY POINTS

- Cell and gene therapy for degenerative diseases of the joints and the spine is a promising area of research with significant potential for clinical development.
- Advances in biotechnology are likely to have a positive impact on tissue engineering and regenerative treatments for the spine.
- However, researchers developing cell and gene therapies for the spine will need to accept the harsh reality that primary, aged, and senescent cells will possess feeble regenerative properties.
- Regenerative medicine and tissue engineering strategies for the spine should therefore consider the use of stem cells combined with mammalian protein production platforms to drive the production of therapeutic proteins and proanabolic growth factors.
- Protein production tools are essential for faster progress in cellular therapy.

INTRODUCTION

Degenerative changes in the intervertebral disc (IVD) cause the loss of normal spine structure and function.[1] IVD degeneration is not typically due to a specific injury but rather it is related to aging. It is possible that injuries can influence the long-term course of spine degeneration. However, spine degeneration is a biomechanically related continuum of molecular, biochemical, cellular, and anatomic alterations evolving over time, due to external insults, such as mechanical or

Disclosure: The authors declare no competing interests.
Financial Support and Sponsorship: See last page of the article.
[a] Department of Regenerative Medicine, State Research Institute Centre for Innovative Medicine, Santariskiu 5, Vilnius 08661, Lithuania; [b] Research Unit of Medical Imaging, Physics and Technology, Faculty of Medicine, University of Oulu, PO Box 5000, Oulu FI-90014, Finland; [c] Centre for Sport, Exercise and Osteoarthritis Research Versus Arthritis, Queen's Medical Centre, Nottingham, UK; [d] King Abdulaziz University, Jeddah, Kingdom of Saudi Arabia; [e] Division of Cell Matrix Biology and Regenerative Medicine, School of Biological Sciences, Faculty of Biology, Medicine and Health, University of Manchester, Manchester Academic Health Sciences Centre, Oxford Road, Manchester, UK
* Corresponding author. Department of Regenerative Medicine, State Research Institute Centre for Innovative Medicine, Santariskiu 5, Vilnius 08661, Lithuania.
E-mail addresses: ali.mobasheri@imcentras.lt; ali.mobasheri@oulu.fi; ali.mobasheri.manuscripts@gmail.com

Neurosurg Clin N Am 31 (2020) 131–139
https://doi.org/10.1016/j.nec.2019.08.015

metabolic injury.[2] Human beings are living longer lives and expect to enjoy pain-free mobile lifestyles. Degenerative diseases of the joints and the spine are largely associated with aging, obesity, poor diets, and occupational factors. Although our ancestors have been around for about 6 million years, modern humans (Homo sapiens) only evolved about 200,000 years ago. Early humans did not live long enough to suffer from age-related musculoskeletal conditions, and degenerative diseases of the joints and the spine are thought to have been extremely rare in early humans, but this is probably because of an underrepresentation of older adults in the skeletal records of the ancient civilizations. Longer life expectancy and the strains, sprains, and overuse of the back over many decades result in a gradual IVD degeneration in the spine.[3] According to the World Health Organization, low back pain (LBP) is a leading cause of disability across the world.[a] LBP occurs in similar proportions in all cultures, interferes with quality of life and work performance, and is currently the most common reason for medical consultations globally. Although LBP has many causes, IVD degeneration has been shown to be an important underlying cause.[4]

Despite the growing prevalence and burden of LBP, IVD, and spine degeneration, there are no effective cures. Degenerative changes in the spine are associated with biomechanical and metabolic alterations and it has been proposed that the degeneration is an adaptation, rather than a disease.[2] It has also been proposed that in the absence of a cure for LBP, IVD, and spine degeneration, the only way to reduce the global burden of these conditions is developing earlier diagnostics, improving management regimes, and conceiving realistic long-term strategies for prevention. Diagnosis of all degenerative joint and spine conditions begins with radiography. However, MRI is increasingly used to image discs, nerves, and the spinal canal space. Computed tomography may be used to resolve inconsistencies between the MRI and the patient's symptoms. Disc studies, also known as discograms, may be ordered to determine if a patient's pain is being caused by a damaged spinal disc. Treatment depends on the type and severity of the patient's condition. In most cases, nonsurgical treatment is all that is required. These treatments may include exercise to increase flexibility and muscle strength, braces, or medication. Pain medication and steroids may be administered via epidural injection. In extreme cases surgery may be required for herniated discs or spinal stenosis, particularly where there is radicular pain. The treatment applied is often for radiculopathy, that is, sciatica, or other nerve issues that cause loss of function, rather than for the LBP itself. In addition to age, gender, lifestyle, and genetic predisposition, other inciting risk factors for disc degeneration may include previous spine injuries or even osteoporosis (**Fig. 1**). This article focuses on IVD degeneration and how cell and gene therapy may be used for spine regeneration.

THE HALLMARKS OF SPINE DEGENERATION

All human diseases are characterized by "hallmarks," which summarize the key biological alterations that occur in a particular disease. For example, cancer comprises 6 biological capabilities that are gradually acquired during the multistep development of human tumors.[5,6] In the case of spine degeneration, there are many similarities with the hallmarks of aging.[7] The hallmarks of aging include genomic instability, telomere attrition, epigenetic alterations, loss of proteostasis, deregulated nutrient sensing, mitochondrial dysfunction, cellular senescence, stem cell exhaustion, and altered intercellular communication. Many of the hallmarks of aging are also seen in IVD degeneration and in articular cartilage in degenerative joint diseases such as osteoarthritis (OA).

CELLULAR SENESCENCE

Senescence of the cells in the specialized tissues of the IVD is a normal part of aging[8]; however, cellular senescence has been shown to be accelerated in degeneration[9] with a range of causes proposed.[10] There is a gradual decline in cell number in the IVD with aging through increased apoptosis, and secondary necrosis reduces the cellularity of the tissue and its ability to repair and regenerate. However, there are reports that there is also increased cellularity in some areas of degenerate discs, with clusters of chondrocyte-like cells forming by cell proliferation in degenerating areas.[11] Interestingly, regional chondrocyte hypocellularity and cloning is also seen in degenerating articular cartilage,[12,13] reminding us of the many similarities between IVD and cartilage, especially with regard to extracellular matrix (ECM) composition.

Changes in cellularity are important because they alter the nutritional status and metabolic substrate requirements of the disc and impact on the

---

[a]https://www.who.int/bulletin/volumes/81/9/Ehrlich.pdf.

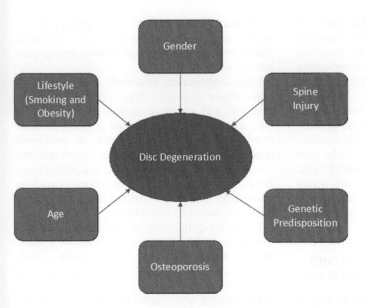

Fig. 1. Risk factors for spine degeneration.

concentration gradients of nutrients, metabolites, and waste products.[11] The normally avascular disc in the healthy adult can become increasingly vascularized and innervated with degeneration and disease. This may lead to an increased supply of oxygen and nutrients to the disc, altering the metabolism of the disc and the phenotype of its resident cells. Furthermore, vascularization and innervation can also introduce other cell types, including inflammatory cells, and a range of bioactive molecules such as proinflammatory cytokines and growth factors. The increased production and secretion of proinflammatory cytokines, particularly tumor necrosis factor α and interleukin 1 β, drives autophagic changes as well as cell death.[14] The relationship between autophagy, apoptosis,[15,16] cell senescence,[17,18] and mitochondrial dysfunction has not been extensively explored in the aging and degenerating disc, and it has been suggested that all these mechanisms are implicated in spine degeneration. Senescent cells cannot divide and they promote the development of a senescence-associated secretory phenotype (SASP). Research at the intersection between the fields of oncology and immunology has demonstrated that the acquisition of SASP can turn senescent stromal fibroblasts into proinflammatory cells that have the ability to promote tumor progression.[19] So what is the relevance of this phenomenon to degenerative diseases of the joints and the spine? SASP defines the ability of senescent cells to express and secrete a variety of extracellular modulators that includes cytokines, chemokines, proteases, growth factors, and bioactive lipids. The SASP secretome can mediate chronic inflammation and stimulate the growth and survival of aggressive and persistent cells with inflammatory potential.[20] SASP may reduce the disc's ability to generate new cells to replace cells lost to necrosis or apoptosis and may seriously compromise the most promising and evidence-based strategies for spine regeneration, including approaches that might use stem cells and gene therapy. Therefore, all future therapeutic and regenerative strategies must first attenuate and eliminate SASP and promote a microenvironment that is more conducive to supporting endogenous or stem cell–facilitated tissue repair and regeneration.[21,22]

MOLECULAR ALTERATIONS IN DISC DEGENERATION

The precise sequence of molecular events involved in the degeneration of the IVD is not clear. However, it is generally accepted that disc degeneration begins at the molecular level early in life, long before the appearance of any radiographic changes or pain symptoms. The degeneration involves a cascade of changes at the cellular and molecular level that results in degradation of the disc ECM, leading to biomechanical failure of this unique and complex structure.[23] IVD degeneration is thought to occur where there is a loss of homeostatic balance with a predominantly catabolic metabolic profile.[24] Once again, similar molecular mechanisms occur in joint degeneration in OA, starting with a long-lasting and asymptomatic "molecular phase," which is followed many years later by loss of articular cartilage, evident radiographic changes, and the appearance of symptoms.[25] Therefore, it is crucially important to understand the implications and potential impact of SASP on the efficacy of regenerative treatments and how SASP might influence the viability, metabolism, and behavior of implanted cells. It is also essential to consider the microenvironmental changes that occur with degeneration. These alterations such as decreases in oxygen, glucose, pH, and changes in osmolarity and loading are likely to influence implanted cells. These important aspects are beyond the scope of this review but they are relevant to cell-injection strategies for IVD regeneration and discussed in detail in these reviews.[22,26]

BIOLOGICAL AND CELLULAR APPROACHES FOR INTERVERTEBRAL DISC REGENERATION

Disease modifications in IVD and cartilage degeneration are extremely challenging and many existing treatments are ineffective. Progress in drug development has been painfully slow compared with other arthritic and rheumatic diseases, especially those with a more prominent inflammatory nature, including rheumatoid arthritis. Recent advances in biological therapy for disc regeneration have particularly been focusing on the nucleus pulposus (NP). This is important because the NP region of the IVD gives the tissue its unique load-bearing properties. The current approaches include using biomaterials, stem cells, and gene vectors. Stem cell–mediated cell therapy has the potential to restore the function and structure of the NP.[27] Viral or nonviral vectors encoding functional genes may potentially generate a therapeutic effect when they are introduced into grafted cells or native cells in the NP. Biomaterial scaffolds may generate a temporally permissive microenvironment for supporting cell division and new tissue growth, allowing the remodeling of scaffolds in the regeneration process.[27] Biomaterial scaffolds may also provide structural support for NP regeneration and serve as a carrier for stem cell and gene vector delivery, while also protecting cells and serving as a reservoir for growth factors. However, as stated earlier, as the disc degenerates, there is decreased cellularity, at least initially. Furthermore, the nutrient supply decreases as the degeneration progresses, thereby limiting cell activity and viability. Therefore, there is a close relationship between cellularity, cell activity, and nutritional support for tissue regeneration.[28] Current biological approaches are likely to place additional demands on an already precarious nutrient supply, and this loss of nutrients associated with disc degeneration may limit the effectiveness of biological and stem cell approaches. Therefore, disc nutrition and spine regeneration are mutually interdependent.

Disc degeneration essentially involves loss of homeostatic control. The balance between anabolic and catabolic activity is disturbed in disc degeneration and normal physiologic turnover of ECM macromolecules is perturbed (**Fig. 2**). New biological therapies must address the imbalance between catabolic and anabolic activity in order to halt disease progression. New treatments must also have the capacity to positively influence IVD metabolism.

Considering the loss of homeostatic control mechanisms, the attenuation of anabolic activity, and the elevation of catabolic processes, greater efforts must be made to stimulate anabolic activity for effective spine regeneration. This is one of the main reasons why current therapeutic strategies are now focusing on the development of cell and gene therapy and recombinant anabolic growth factors. There is significant ongoing effort in this area, especially focusing on the use of stem cells and the application of chondrocyte and stem cell–derived growth factors.

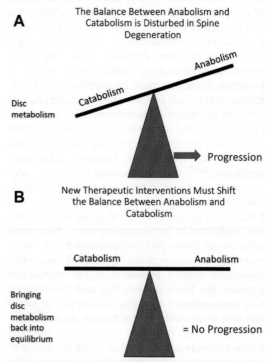

Fig. 2. (*A*) Loss of the delicate physiologic balance between anabolism and catabolism in disc degeneration leads to impaired disc metabolism and disease progression. (*B*) Effective drugs can bring disc metabolism back into equilibrium and attenuate the rate of disease progression.

One crucial quantum leap in the development of new therapies for degenerative diseases of the joint has been the realization and acceptance that the most ideal treatments must target the affected joint through injection, directly targeting the compromised structures. The same basic concept applies to the IVD. However, many of the key researchers in this field have yet to accept that biological therapy, whether using autologous cells and stem cells, cannot be achieved with primary tissue-derived native cells. Primary and native cells do not possess the necessary regenerative attributes. Despite progress and advancements in mesenchymal stem cell (MSC) biology and the introduction of various bioactive scaffolds and growth factors in preclinical studies, current clinical trials are still at early stages with preliminary aims to evaluate safety, feasibility, and efficacy,[29,30] and this is where we must focus our efforts. Strategies that potentiate endogenous IVD disc progenitors may offer a valid alternative to the exogenous cell transplantation but new clinical trials need to be designed and carried out to make this important comparison.

Clinical trials of cell therapies, and MSCs in particular, have so far demonstrated only limited efficacy. A company called DiscGenics is about to start trials of a healthy donor NP cell therapy for IVD degeneration.[b] Although we anxiously wait for outcomes of several ongoing stem cell trials, there are several pharmaceutical companies that have innovated in this area of cell and gene therapy by focusing efforts on developing treatments using mammalian protein production platforms, including transformed and modified cells, as well as immortalized cells that were originally developed as research tools and protein packaging cell lines for overproduction of target proteins. Biotechnology has already offered us powerful and versatile tools for the overproduction of therapeutic proteins. We need to accept the fact that new therapeutic innovations for degenerative diseases of the joints and the spine may come from other biological and biomedical disciplines, including biotechnology, protein engineering, and immunology.

MAMMALIAN PROTEIN PRODUCTION PLATFORMS

Mammalian protein production platforms are cell factories that are used for large-scale production of antibodies and therapeutic proteins.[31] Expression of proteins in mammalian cells is an enabling technology that is vitally important for many functional studies on human and higher eukaryotic genes. Mammalian cell expression systems allow the production of proteins, especially of those of clinical relevance and human origin.[32] Over the last few decades these platforms have evolved and had a profound impact on many areas of basic and applied research, and an increasing number of biological drugs are now recombinant mammalian proteins made using these tools.[33] Recombinant proteins and antibodies are now produced in mammalian cell lines instead of bacterial expression systems to ensure that proper protein folding and posttranslational modifications, which are essential for full biological activity, are properly introduced in not only a eukaryotic but also a "mammalian" context.

Mammalian cell expression systems are the dominant tools for producing complex biotherapeutic proteins.[34] The most commonly used mammalian cell lines found in the research and industrial therapeutic protein production settings are Chinese hamster ovary cells (CHO)[35] and human embryonic kidney 293 cells (HEK-293).[36] Various mammalian and nonmammalian expression systems are also being used for protein and glycoprotein production, and recent cellular engineering strategies have been developed to increase protein and glycoprotein productivity.[37] "Omics" technologies are continually being used to improve cellular expression systems and enhance such platforms for therapeutic protein production. **Fig. 3** summarizes the expression systems used for protein and glycoprotein production by industry.

Transient expression systems in mammalian cells have also become the method of choice for producing large quantities of antibodies.[38] The ability to scale-up allows biotechnology companies to produce sufficient quantities of therapeutic antibodies and proteins for tests in preclinical studies and conducting early phase clinical trials. Without such tools, progress in biological and cellular therapy would grind to a halt.

PLATFORMS FOR OVERPRODUCTION OF RECOMBINANT GROWTH FACTORS

Production of large quantities of a growth factor capable of stimulating tissue repair and new ECM synthesis will require mammalian cell models that truly mimic chondrocytes or NP cells, with phenotypic chondrocytic and NP-like properties. However, there are no such cellular tools for use in this context. However, other cellular models are

---

[b]https://www.prnewswire.com/news-releases/discgenics-announces-first-patient-treated-in-us-clinical-trial-of-idct-for-degenerative-disc-disease-300636859.html.

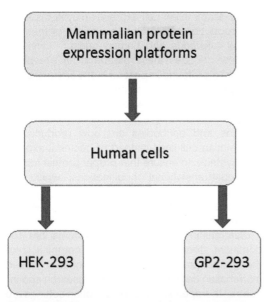

Fig. 3. Expression systems used for human protein and glycoprotein production by biopharmaceutical industries. (*Adapted from* Lalonde M-E, Durocher Y. Therapeutic glycoprotein production in mammalian cells. J. Biotechnol. 2017;251:129; with permission.)

available, including CHO, HEK-293 cells, and their derivatives such as GP2-293. These are immortalized cell lines that function as "cellular factories" for overproduction of proteins. GP2-293 cells are specialized protein packaging cells. These cells are specialized transfection models, protein packaging tools for overproduction of target human proteins, and are promising candidates for overproducing therapeutic proteins and growth factors that native primary cells (ie, chondrocytes, NP cells) or stem cells (ie, MSCs) cannot produce in sufficiently large quantities, either in the short term or in the long term. Although these cells cannot be used in their immortalized form for the development of clinically relevant cell therapies for the joints and the spine, they can be irradiated to obliterate their proliferation capacity so that they remain protein packaging cellular factories, but lose the ability to proliferate. Elimination of their proliferation capacity through irradiation makes the use of such cells feasible in cellular therapies, especially if the cells are to be injected into the closed microenvironment of the synovial joint or the IVD, where they will be isolated from the circulatory system. Irradiated cells will retain their capacity for protein overproduction, but they cannot divide and proliferate, which means that they will

die several days after being injected into the joint or the spine. Of course there are alternative approaches to using cells. Microparticles have been developed for controlled growth differentiation factor 6 (GDF6) delivery to direct adipose stem cell–based NP regeneration. Effective encapsulation and controlled delivery of recombinant human GDF6 has been shown to maintain its activity and induced ASC differentiation to NP cells and synthesis of an NP-like matrix. Microparticles may therefore be suitable for controlled growth factor release in regenerative strategies for treatment of IVD degeneration.[39] However, transformed cells and protein production platforms have the potential for controlled and sustained growth factor synthesis and release over a period of days.

PRODUCTION OF TRANSFORMING GROWTH FACTOR β1 (TGF-β1) BY PROTEIN PACKAGING CELLS GP2-293 IN THE KOLON TissueGenes CELL AND GENE THERAPY PRODUCT—INVOSSA

Invossa[c] is a unique first-in-class cell and gene therapy targeting knee OA through a single intraarticular injection of joint-derived chondrocytes, irradiated GP2-293, and, most importantly, the biological growth factors that they overproduce to possibly promote anabolic repair and regeneration in the diseased joint as a future possibility in the treatment of OA. The same scientific principle may be applied to the degenerated disc (**Fig. 4**A), where TGF-β could be replaced by a more appropriate growth factor such as GDF6.[40] Therefore, a more suitable growth factor such as GDF6 can be overproduced instead.

If regenerating the NP region is desired, native patient-derived NP cells will not have the capacity to overproduce an anabolic growth factor in sufficiently high quantities for successful cellular therapy and regenerative applications. Human GP2-293 cells are one of the key components of Invossa and carry out the vital function of overproducing the crucially important growth factor; hence they offer an attractive alternative for IVD regeneration strategies. GP2-293 cells have been used throughout the whole developmental process for Invossa, from the first production of the Master Cell Bank to the next step, which is the development of the working cell bank and the final product formulation. As mentioned earlier, GP2-293 is an HEK-293–based retroviral packaging cell line used for large-scale protein

---

[c]Kolon TissueGene (KTG) is a US based company and they have TG-C in clinical trials. Kolon Life Sciences (KLS) is based in Korea and they have the marketed product Invossa-K. If approved in the United States, KTG will have Invossa in the United States.

A **General Concept for Invossa Applied to The Disc**

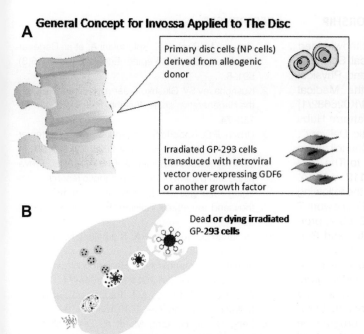

Primary disc cells (NP cells) derived from alleogenic donor

Irradiated GP-293 cells transduced with retroviral vector over-expressing GDF6 or another growth factor

B

Dead **or dying irradiated** GP-**293 cells**

Phagocytosis by spine **resident macrophages**

Fig. 4. (*A*) The intraarticular injection concept for Invossa, originally developed as a novel cell and gene therapy targeting knee OA, can be modified and repurposed for IVD regeneration. In this concept injection of primary NP cells or stem cells and irradiated GP2-293 overproduce a suitable growth factor, such as GDF6. This is the biological growth factor that is thought to promote the anabolic repair and regeneration of IVD. Alternatively GDF6 could be used with any other growth factor or combination of growth factors as the field of IVD regeneration progresses. (*B*) Phagocytosis and destruction of dead GP2-293 or their cellular debris by spine resident macrophages.

production. It is a cellular platform for overproduction of therapeutically relevant human proteins. This is the first time that such a human protein production platform has been used in the context of OA treatment and cartilage regeneration. It is conceivable that the same approach may work for the IVD, whether with TGFβ or GDF6 or an alternative growth factor, as these cells can function as a protein-producing tool and "cellular factory" for therapeutic growth factors that can target degenerative pathways in IVD.

SAFETY OF GP2-293 CELLS IN INVOSSA

Transduced and irradiated GP2-293 cells may be transformed triploid cells but they have lost their capacity for proliferation through irradiation. Therefore, the GP2-293 cells in Invossa cannot survive and proliferate in the joint or in the spine. It is envisaged that these cells will simply carry out their transient function as radiation inactivated transfection models, protein packaging tools, and "cellular factories" for overproduction of therapeutic growth factors such as TGF-β1. Therefore, the cells cannot survive for more than a very short period of days after being injected into the joint or the spine. After the cells carry out their TGF-β1 production duties, they will die and their remains will be cleared by joint resident inflammatory macrophages through the process of phagocytosis (**Fig. 4B**).

The scientific basis for the use of mammalian cell transfection models in new cell-based

therapies for the spine is clear in the development of Invossa. There is a well-established literature on the use of HEK-293 cells as a transfection model and cell culture model for protein production in a research setting but there is potential to extend this concept to clinically relevant biological therapies. The efficacy and safety of HEK-293 cells and their derivatives in cell therapy has not been extensively investigated but the prospects for future use of transfection tools in regenerative medicine is very positive, especially because native and untransformed cells do not have the appropriate regenerative capacity.

SUMMARY

Cell and gene therapy for degenerative diseases of the joint and spine is a promising area of research with significant potential for clinical development. However, there are currently no effective treatments for spine degeneration. The significant recent advances in the field of biotechnology are likely to have a positive impact on tissue engineering and regenerative treatments for the spine. We need to accept the harsh reality that primary, aged, and senescent cells are unlikely to possess robust regenerative properties. Regenerative medicine and tissue engineering strategies for the spine should consider the use of stem cells combined with mammalian protein production platforms to drive the production of therapeutic proteins and growth factors.

FINANCIAL SUPPORT AND SPONSORSHIP

Funding for S.M. Richardson is acknowledged from the Biotechnology and Biological Sciences Research Council; the Engineering and Physical Sciences Research Council; and the Medical Research Council [grant number MR/K026682/1] via the UK Regenerative Medicine Platform Hubs "Acellular Approaches for Therapeutic Delivery", as well as the Medical Research Council via a Confidence-in-Concept 2014 award to The University of Manchester (MC_PC_14112 v.2). A. Mobasheri has received funding from the following sources: The European Commission Framework 7 programme (EU FP7; HEALTH.2012.2.4.5-2, project number 305815; Novel Diagnostics and Biomarkers for Early Identification of Chronic Inflammatory Joint Diseases). The Innovative Medicines Initiative Joint Undertaking under grant agreement No. 115770, resources of which are composed of financial contribution from the European Union's Seventh Framework programme (FP7/2007-2013) and EFPIA companies' in-kind contribution. The author also wishes to acknowledge funding from the European Commission through a Marie Curie Intra-European Fellowship for Career Development grant (project number 625746; acronym: CHONDRION; FP7-PEOPLE-2013-IEF). A. Mobasheri also wishes to acknowledge financial support from the European Structural and Social Funds (ES Struktūrinès Paramos) through the Research Council of Lithuania (Lietuvos Mokslo Taryba) according to the activity 'Improvement of researchers' qualification by implementing world-class R&D projects' of Measure No. 09.3.3-LMT-K-712 (grant application code: 09.3.3-LMT-K-712-01-0157, agreement No. DOTSUT-215) and the new funding programme: Attracting Foreign Researchers for Research Implementation (2018-2022) [grant No 0.2.2-LMTK-718-02-0022]. The author has received payments from King Abdulaziz University, Jeddah, Kingdom of Saudi Arabia. The author also declares that he has consulted for the following companies in the last three years: Abbvie, Aché Laboratórios Farmacêuticos S.A., AlphaSights, Galapagos, Guidepoint Global, Kolon TissueGene, Pfizer Consumer Health (PCH), Servier, Bioiberica S.A. and Science Branding Communications.

ACKNOWLEDGMENTS

Soraya Mobasheri provided the original digital artwork in **Fig. 4**A and Roxana Mobasheri provided the original digital artwork in **Fig. 4**B.

REFERENCES

1. Gallucci M, Puglielli E, Splendiani A, et al. Degenerative disorders of the spine. Eur Radiol 2005;15(3): 591–8.
2. Kushchayev SV, Glushko T, Jarraya M, et al. ABCs of the degenerative spine. Insights Imaging 2018;9(2): 253–74.
3. Urban JPG, Roberts S. Degeneration of the intervertebral disc. Arthritis Res Ther 2003;5(3):120–30.
4. Cheung KMC, Karppinen J, Chan D, et al. Prevalence and pattern of lumbar magnetic resonance imaging changes in a population study of one thousand forty-three individuals. Spine 2009;34(9): 934–40.
5. Hanahan D, Weinberg RA. The hallmarks of cancer. Cell 2000;100(1):57–70.
6. Hanahan D, Weinberg RA. Hallmarks of cancer: the next generation. Cell 2011;144(5):646–74.
7. López-Otín C, Blasco MA, Partridge L, et al. The hallmarks of aging. Cell 2013;153(6):1194–217.
8. Feng C, Liu H, Yang M, et al. Disc cell senescence in intervertebral disc degeneration: Causes and molecular pathways. Cell Cycle 2016;15(13): 1674–84.
9. Le Maitre CL, Freemont AJ, Hoyland JA. Accelerated cellular senescence in degenerate intervertebral discs: a possible role in the pathogenesis of intervertebral disc degeneration. Arthritis Res Ther 2007;9(3):R45.
10. Patil P, Niedernhofer LJ, Robbins PD, et al. Cellular senescence in intervertebral disc aging and degeneration. Curr Mol Biol Rep 2018;4(4):180–90.
11. Roberts S. Disc morphology in health and disease. Biochem Soc Trans 2002;30(Pt 6):864–9.
12. Martin JA, Buckwalter JA. Aging, articular cartilage chondrocyte senescence and osteoarthritis. Biogerontology 2002;3(5):257–64.
13. Martin JA, Buckwalter JA. Human chondrocyte senescence and osteoarthritis. Biorheology 2002; 39(1–2):145–52.
14. Gruber HE, Hoelscher GL, Ingram JA, et al. Autophagy in the degenerating human intervertebral disc: in vivo molecular and morphological evidence, and induction of autophagy in cultured annulus cells exposed to proinflammatory cytokines-implications for disc degeneration. Spine 2015;40(11):773–82.
15. Ding F, Shao Z, Xiong L. Cell death in intervertebral disc degeneration. Apoptosis 2013;18(7):777–85.
16. Zhao C-Q, Jiang L-S, Dai L-Y. Programmed cell death in intervertebral disc degeneration. Apoptosis 2006;11(12):2079–88.
17. Gruber HE, Ingram JA, Norton HJ, et al. Senescence in cells of the aging and degenerating intervertebral disc: immunolocalization of senescence-associated beta-galactosidase in human and sand rat discs. Spine 2007;32(3):321–7.

18. Kim K-W, Chung H-N, Ha K-Y, et al. Senescence mechanisms of nucleus pulposus chondrocytes in human intervertebral discs. Spine J 2009;9(8):658–66.

19. Coppé J-P, Desprez P-Y, Krtolica A, et al. The senescence-associated secretory phenotype: the dark side of tumor suppression. Annu Rev Pathol 2010;5:99–118.

20. Lopes-Paciencia S, Saint-Germain E, Rowell M-C, et al. The senescence-associated secretory phenotype and its regulation. Cytokine 2019;117:15–22.

21. Richardson SM, Hoyland JA, Mobasheri R, et al. Mesenchymal stem cells in regenerative medicine: opportunities and challenges for articular cartilage and intervertebral disc tissue engineering. J Cell Physiol 2010;222(1):23–32.

22. Richardson SM, Kalamegam G, Pushparaj PN, et al. Mesenchymal stem cells in regenerative medicine: Focus on articular cartilage and intervertebral disc regeneration. Methods 2016;99:69–80.

23. Anderson DG, Tannoury C. Molecular pathogenic factors in symptomatic disc degeneration. Spine J 2005;5(6 Suppl):260S–6S.

24. Kadow T, Sowa G, Vo N, et al. Molecular basis of intervertebral disc degeneration and herniations: what are the important translational questions? Clin Orthop Relat Res 2015;473(6):1903–12.

25. Kraus VB, Blanco FJ, Englund M, et al. Call for standardized definitions of osteoarthritis and risk stratification for clinical trials and clinical use. Osteoarthr Cartil 2015;23(8):1233–41.

26. Sakai D, Andersson GBJ. Stem cell therapy for intervertebral disc regeneration: obstacles and solutions. Nat Rev Rheumatol 2015;11(4):243–56.

27. Priyadarshani P, Li Y, Yao L. Advances in biological therapy for nucleus pulposus regeneration. Osteoarthr Cartil 2016;24(2):206–12.

28. Huang Y-C, Urban JPG, Luk KDK. Intervertebral disc regeneration: do nutrients lead the way? Nat Rev Rheumatol 2014;10(9):561–6.

29. Lee WY-W, Wang B. Cartilage repair by mesenchymal stem cells: clinical trial update and perspectives. J Orthop Translat 2017;9:76–88.

30. Sun Y, Leung VY, Cheung KM. Clinical trials of intervertebral disc regeneration: current status and future developments. Int Orthop 2019;43(4):1003–10.

31. Zucchelli S, Patrucco L, Persichetti F, et al. Engineering translation in mammalian cell factories to increase protein yield: the unexpected use of long non-coding SINEUP RNAs. Comput Struct Biotechnol J 2016;14:404–10.

32. Aricescu AR, Owens RJ. Expression of recombinant glycoproteins in mammalian cells: towards an integrative approach to structural biology. Curr Opin Struct Biol 2013;23(3):345–56.

33. Bandaranayake AD, Almo SC. Recent advances in mammalian protein production. FEBS Lett 2014;588(2):253–60.

34. Estes S, Melville M. Mammalian cell line developments in speed and efficiency. Adv Biochem Eng Biotechnol 2014;139:11–33.

35. Omasa T, Onitsuka M, Kim W-D. Cell engineering and cultivation of chinese hamster ovary (CHO) cells. Curr Pharm Biotechnol 2010;11(3):233–40.

36. Dyson MR. Fundamentals of expression in mammalian cells. Adv Exp Med Biol 2016;896:217–24.

37. Lalonde M-E, Durocher Y. Therapeutic glycoprotein production in mammalian cells. J Biotechnol 2017;251:128–40.

38. Vink T, Oudshoorn-Dickmann M, Roza M, et al. A simple, robust and highly efficient transient expression system for producing antibodies. Methods 2014;65(1):5–10.

39. Hodgkinson T, Stening JZ, White LJ, et al. Microparticles for controlled growth differentiation factor 6 delivery to direct adipose stem cell-based nucleus pulposus regeneration. J Tissue Eng Regen Med 2019. https://doi.org/10.1002/term.2882.

40. Clarke LE, McConnell JC, Sherratt MJ, et al. Growth differentiation factor 6 and transforming growth factor-beta differentially mediate mesenchymal stem cell differentiation, composition, and micromechanical properties of nucleus pulposus constructs. Arthritis Res Ther 2014;16(2):R67.

Emerging Percutaneous Ablative and Radiosurgical Techniques for Treatment of Spinal Metastases

Muhamed Hadzipasic, MD, PhD[a], Alexandra M. Giantini-Larsen, MD[b],
Claudio E. Tatsui, MD[c], John H. Shin, MD[a],*

KEYWORDS

- Interstitial thermal therapy (LITT) • Radiofrequency ablation (RFA) • Cryoablation
- Stereotactic radiosurgery (SRS)

KEY POINTS

- A range of minimally invasive techniques exists for the treatment of metastatic spinal disease.
- Efficacy of minimally invasive techniques has not yet been rigorously tested but early results are promising.
- The future of spinal oncology likely will depend on multidisciplinary input and integration of a range of techniques tailored for the specific malignancy and involved anatomy.

INTRODUCTION

Metastatic spinal disease occurs in 40% to 50% of patients with cancer and is a common cause of pain, disability, and morbidity. Hence, medical and surgical approaches strive to preserve or restore neurologic function, relieve pain, and stabilize the spine. As systemic therapies for metastatic cancer evolve with the introduction of novel targeted therapies, increasing overall survival necessitates the need for optimization of strategies to achieve local control of disease in the spine, epidural space, and surrounding tissues. The goal in the care for patients with spinal metastases is to relieve the pain and disability from nerve and spinal cord compression, while limiting the treatment related morbidity so that these patients can live to reap the benefits of intervention.

Percutaneous ablative and stereotactic radiosurgery (SRS) have emerged as less-invasive methods to treat spinal metastases compared with traditional open surgical approaches. These interventions add to the current armamentarium of conventional open surgery, minimally invasive percutaneous stabilization, cement augmentation, and conventional radiotherapy (CRT). Although patients with metastatic disease to the spine may meet clinical criteria for open conventional surgery based on the assessment of their pain, neurology, mechanical spine stability, and cancer type, not every patient is a suitable candidate due to overall health status and concern for the magnitude of intervention.

Disclosure Statement: The authors have nothing to disclose.
[a] Department of Neurosurgery, Massachusetts General Hospital, Harvard Medical School, 55 Fruit Street, Boston, MA 02114, USA; [b] Department of Neurological Surgery, New York-Presbyterian Hospital/Weill Cornell Medical Center, 525 East 68 Street, Box 99, New York, NY 10065, USA; [c] Department of Neurosurgery, Division of Surgery, The University of Texas MD Anderson Cancer Center, 1515 Holcombe Boulevard, Houston, TX 77030, USA
* Corresponding author.
E-mail address: shin.john@mgh.harvard.edu

neurosurgery.theclinics.com

The goal of the evolving percutaneous ablative and radiosurgical techniques is to improve function, decrease pain, and control local spread of disease with much lower risk to the patient than a traditional surgical approach to the metastatic lesion. These techniques can be used in combination with surgery as well as other minimally invasive techniques, such as vertebral augmentation, including kyphoplasty and vertebroplasty, to help provide local tumor control as well as palliation.

This article reviews emerging percutaneous ablative and radiosurgical techniques for treatment of spinal metastases. The percutaneous ablative techniques discussed are laser interstitial thermal therapy (LITT), radiofrequency ablation (RFA), and cryoablation. SRS also is reviewed as an adjuvant to surgical resection or separation surgery.

ABLATIVE TECHNIQUES
Laser Interstitial Thermal Therapy

LITT is a minimally invasive therapy that utilizes a laser to deliver thermal ablation to tumor cells. This therapy has been used in both the brain and spine to deliver precise thermal ablation to tumors. Within the brain, a main advantage of the technique is the ability to access tumors that are difficult to access surgically due to anatomic location and proximity to eloquent areas. Other advantages include the minimally invasive nature of the surgery and quick recovery from treatment experienced by patients.

This therapy has recently been pioneered in the treatment of metastatic tumors to the spine. Tatsui and colleagues[1] first reported the use of spinal LITT for the management of spinal metastasis as an alternative to separation surgery in 2015. With this technique, a laser is directed under magnetic resonance imaging (MRI) guidance to the area of the tumor.[1–3] Intraoperative thermal MRI is then used to monitor heat delivered to the tumor as well as surrounding tissue.[4]

In this first study of 11 patients, there was significant decrease in mean thickness of the epidural tumor as well as a significant reduction in degree of epidural spinal cord compression after treatment compared with before treatment. In addition, patients reported decreased pain and increased quality of life after treatment. All patients in study received stereotactic spine radiosurgery (SSRS) after LITT, and further studies describe LITT as an alternative option to surgery in select patients prior to SSRS.[5]

As discussed by Tatsui and colleagues,[1] this technique allows patients with high degrees of spinal cord compression due to metastatic spinal tumors to receive a targeted therapy to decrease compression and improve function. Although recovery from traditional surgical intervention would delay systemic therapy, often by multiple weeks, LITT can be performed without interruption or delay of systemic therapy.[5] General contraindications to use of this technique include patients who are unable to undergo MRI and those with severe neurologic deficits that require immediate decompression. An example of this therapy in clinical practice is illustrated later.

Case illustration
A 68-year-old woman with widely metastatic alveolar sarcoma presented with refractory right thoracic radicular pain in a T10-T11 distribution. Her systemic disease was progressing and resistant to multiple chemotherapy agents. She had a history of prior CRT to T10 to T12. Her KPS was 70% and neurologic examination at presentation was normal with the exception of sensory polyneuropathy and right thoracic radiculopathy. MRI of the thoracic spine demonstrated tumor involving the left T11 costotransverse joint with significant epidural extension at T10 to T11 and T11 to T12 (**Fig. 1**). Given the extent of systemic disease progression, the patient was receiving a second cycle of anlotinib and was recommended surgical decompression of the spinal cord prior to salvage SSRS.

The patient was bought to the operating room and fiducial markers applied to the region of interest. An MRI-compatible spinous process clamp was applied in proximity to the fiducial markers and covered with a sterile plastic bag (**Fig. 2**A). The MRI coil is held with a plastic cradle to avoid contact with skin and the patient is transferred to the MRI magnet to acquire 1-mm axial cuts in T2 sequence of the region of interest (see **Fig. 2**B). These images are exported to an image guidance system for subsequent surface matching registration of the skin fiducials (see **Fig. 2**C). Once the MRI images are acquired, axial, sagittal and coronal reconstruction is used to plan the trajectory for laser catheter placement. A 10-mm to 12-mm zone of ablation is estimated for each catheter; therefore, multiple trajectories are planned in order to cover the entirety of the epidural tumor (**Fig. 3**).

After registration of the image guidance, the fiducials are removed and the region of interest is prepped with sterile technique. A navigated Jamshidi needle is used to match the planned trajectories. Once the needle reaches its target, it is exchanged to plastic access cannulas. In this example, 9 catheters were used with multiple trajectories. After catheter placement, everything is covered with sterile technique and the patient is

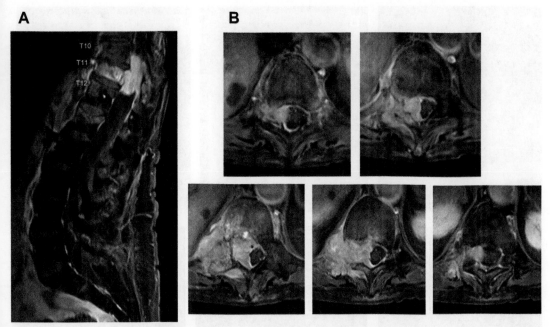

Fig. 1. MRI of the T spine in (*A*) sagittal and (*B*) axial cuts through the thoracic spinal cord, demonstrating the extension of the epidural tumor causing a Bilsky 2° of spinal cord compression. T, thoracic.

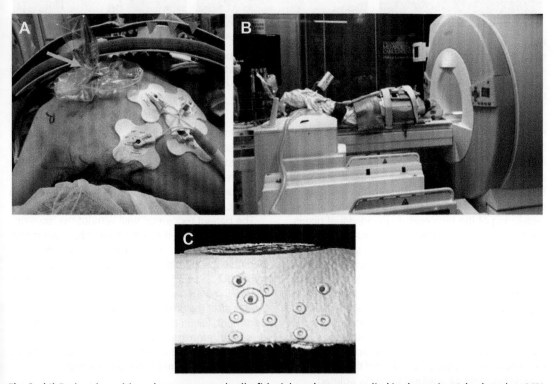

Fig. 2. (*A*) Patient is positioned prone over gel rolls; fiducial markers are applied in the patient's back and an MRI-compatible spinous process clamp is applied with sterile technique and covered with a sterile plastic bag (*arrow*); the MRI coil is subsequently applied over the fiducial markers help by a plastic cradle to avoid contact with the dorsal skin (*arrowheads*). (*B*) Patient is transported to the MRI magnet for obtaining 1-mm axial cuts in T2 sequence of the zone of interest. (*C*) Intraoperative images are uploaded to the navigation system and a 3-dimensional model is developed for surface matching of the fiducial markers.

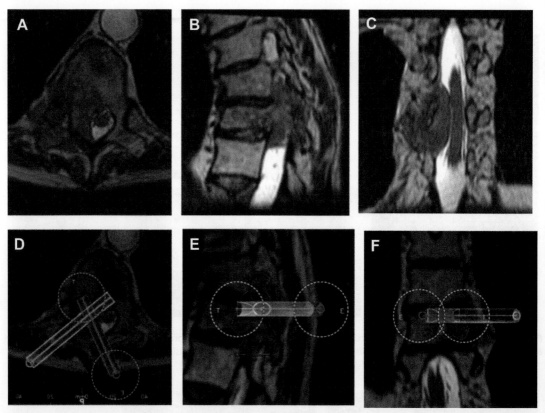

Fig. 3. Intraoperative T2 image of the epidural tumor in (A) axial, (B) sagittal, and (C) coronal view. Images are exported to the image guidance system. After outlining the epidural tumor to be ablated, multiple trajectories are planned in order to proceed with the treatment. Each catheter is considered enough to cover 10 mm to 12 mm of tumor and the authors plan several trajectories in axial (D), sagittal (E), and coronal (F) planes in order to ablate the epidural tumor.

returned to MRI to localize scans in the exact axial plane of each catheter (**Fig. 4**). The laser catheter (Visualase, Medtronic, Minneapolis, MN) is inserted in the first access cannula and MRI thermography is used to estimate the axial distribution of heat in real time. The software allows monitoring of the temperature in individual pixels. Points along the interface of the tumor and the dura mater are selected and an upper limit of 50°C is set; if this temperature is reached, the system automatically deactivates, avoiding thermal damage to the spinal cord and nerve roots (**Fig. 5**). During ablation, the anesthesiologist closely monitors the patient and interrupts the ventilation for approximately 2 minutes. Once this is completed, the laser catheter is moved to the subsequent access cannula and the procedure is repeated until all epidural tumor is ablated.

Once the treatment is completed, a post-treatment MRI image with and without contrast of the region of interest is performed. As the ablated tissue tends to have hyperintense signal in the noncontrast scan, the best way to demonstrate the ablation is to perform subtraction of the non-contrasted images, which outlines the real contrast enhancement. The typical finding is a dark area around the dura, which is easily identifiable due to the enhancement of the epidural veins (**Fig. 6**).

The patient recovered well without the development of motor deficits. She had significant improvement in her thoracic radiculopathy, because the ablation zone included the neuroforamina of T10 to T11 and T11 to T12, acting as a thermal ganglionectomy. She received SSRS 3 days after the procedure and continued systemic treatment. Given the minimally invasive treatment, a spinal stabilization procedure was avoided because collateral damage to posterior elements and to the vertebral body was minimal.

Radiofrequency Ablation

RFA is a percutaneous, minimally invasive technique that uses heat produced by high-frequency alternating current (generally ranging from 300 kHz

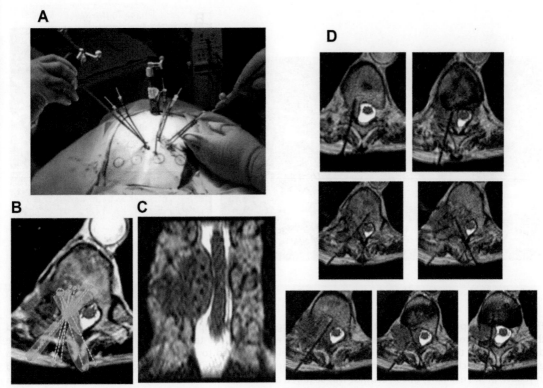

Fig. 4. (*A*) Intraoperative picture illustrating fiber placement. A navigated Jamshidi needle is used to reach the epidural tumor and is exchanged to a plastic access cannula. In this example, several catheters in tandem and in multiple trajectories are used to ablate the epidural tumor. (*B*) Reconstruction in the axial plane demonstrating the planned trajectories for catheter placement. (*C, D*) After appropriate sterile draping, the patient is returned to the MRI scanner and images of verification of each catheter placement are obtained in coronal (*C*) and axial (*D*) planes.

to 600 kHz) to damage tumor cells.[6] An electrode is placed within the target area under image guidance, and the current is passed to the tissue surrounding the electrode. After sufficient heating of the tissue, cell death and coagulation necrosis occur.[7]

Several studies have evaluated the effectiveness of RFA in bony metastases.[8–10] In 2002, Gronemeyer and colleagues[9] published a single-site retrospective review of 10 patients with unresectable spinal metastases in the thoracic spine, lumbar spine, and/or sacrum who received RFA. 90% of patients reported reduced pain using the visual analog scale (VAS), with an average pain reduction of 74.4%. In 2014, a multicenter retrospective review of 92 patients with metastatic spinal lesions who received RFA found that patient-reported pain using VAS was significantly reduced at 1 week, 1 month, and 6 months after the procedure.[8] In terms of pain medication use after the procedure, 54% of patients reported decrease use of pain medication, 30% reported no change in usage, and 16% reported increased usage of pain medication.

RFA is often combined with vertebral augmentation in cases of stable pathologic vertebral compression fractures to help decrease pain and improve function.[11–15] A multicenter retrospective study by Reyes and colleagues[12] looked at the outcomes for 49 individuals with metastatic lesions to the spine who underwent RFA and cement augmentation. RFA and cement augmentation were performed concurrently during the same procedural time. There was a significant reduction in Oswestry Disability Index as well as VAS after the procedure compared with before the procedure. Tumors showed decreased metabolic activity on positron emission tomography as well as decreased tumor volume and enhancing rim on postcontrast MRI after the ablation. There were no major complications reported.

Similarly, Wallace and colleagues[11] retrospectively reviewed 55 cases of spinal metastases that were treated with both RFA and vertebroplasty. At 3-month follow-up, local tumor control of spinal lesions that received RFA was 89% (41/46). Progression of systemic disease was noted in 80% of these

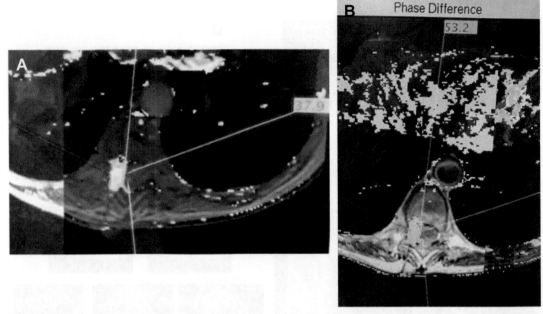

Fig. 5. (*A*) Intraoperative screenshot of the MRI thermography. The temperature is depicted in color gradient and the green lines represent the critical pixels where the authors set the temperature limit in the interface of the dura mater and the tumor. In this example, that pixel is estimated to be at 37.9°C. (*B*) The software outlines each pixel that achieved ablative temperature and generates a model of the predicted area of ablation depicted in yellow. In this example, this screenshot was acquired at the end of the ablation cycle, when the temperature in the critical pixel exceeded the 50°C limit and the system automatically deactivated.

cases (37/46). Of the individuals who had progression of systemic disease, 86% (32/37) still had radiographic control of spinal tumor that received ablation. At 6-month follow-up, local tumor control in the cases overall and those with progression metastatic cancer was 74% (26/35) and 71% (22/31), respectively. At 1-year follow-up, radiographic local tumor control in the cases overall and those with progression metastatic cancer was 70% (21/30) and 67% (18/27), respectively.

RFA alone has been shown to decrease pain and improve function in individuals with

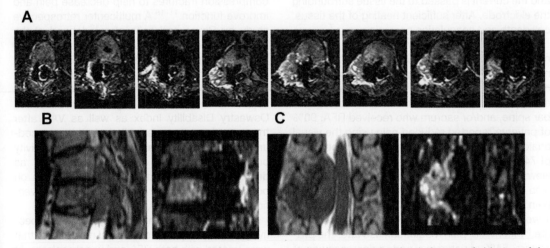

Fig. 6. (*A*) Axial subtraction T1 with and without contrast images demonstrating the dark zone of ablation of the epidural tumor. (*B*, *C*) Sagittal (*B*) and coronal (*C*) images comparing the preoperative extension of the epidural tumor with the respective post-treatment subtraction scan to illustrate the craniocaudal and lateral extension of the ablation volume.

metastatic disease to the spinal cord as well as radiographically decrease tumor size. An advantage of the technique is the ability to concurrently perform vertebral augmentation for individuals with pathologic vertebral compression fractures. These techniques, which can be performed under minimal anesthesia or conscious sedation, may provide pain relief and improvement in function to individuals with metastatic cancer to the spine who are poor surgical candidates due to their health status.

Cryoablation

Cryoablation is a percutaneous, minimally invasive, image-guided technique that uses extreme cold temperatures to kill cells. A cryoprobe is localized to the area of the spinal tumor using image guidance. Either a unipedicular or bipedicular approach can be utilized to access the vertebral body lesion, depending on extent of involvement of the neoplasm within the vertebral body.[6,16] For lesions that involves more than 50% of the vertebral body, a bipedicular approach is recommended for use.[16] Tomasian and colleagues[16] reported in a series of 31 vertebral metastases treated with cryotherapy that each procedure consisted of at least 1 freeze/active thaw/freeze cycle that were 10 minutes, 5 minutes, and 10 minutes, respectively. The freeze phase commonly uses liquid argon to lower the temperature at the cryoprobe tip. An enlarging ice ball forms as the quick cooling of the tip is exchanged with the tissue surrounding the probe.[6,17–19] The freeze and thaw cycles create an osmotic gradient across the cells, which leads to cell membrane injury and cell death.

Preoperatively, the size and location of the tumor are used to determine the number and diameter of cryoprobes used during the procedure.[20] Computed tomography (CT) is used to visualize the effect of cryoablation during the procedure, as the area of damaged tissue forms a hypoattenuating ice ball.[21] Intraoperative CT is helpful in determining the number of freeze/active thaw/freeze cycles required for effective cover of the tumor in the ice ball.[11,16]

Cryoablation is most commonly used in metastatic spinal tumors with a high soft tissue component and is preferred over RFA for osteoblastic lesions, because the thickened bone decreases the effectiveness of the high-frequency alternating current used in RFA.[6] Advantages to cryoablation include the individualized nature of the procedure, including the number and width of probes used as well as number of freeze/active thaw/freeze cycles that are performed. Real-time monitoring of the ice ball formation allows for adjustments to the

number of cycles performed to ensure encapsulation of the entire tumor occurs during the procedure. It is estimated that dependable cell death occurs 3 mm behind the ice ball margin, so encapsulation of tissue immediately outside of the lesion would be required for complete obliteration of the lesion.[22]

STEREOTACTIC SPINE RADIOSURGERY

SSRS has become a key modality in the multimodal treatment of metastatic spinal tumors. The biologic radiologic dose advantage of this form of radiation helps achieve palliation of pain as well as local tumor control for spinal metastases. It can be applied to the spine in various settings, including as (1) standalone therapy; (2) reirradiation after CRT failure, that is, local disease progression; or (3) a postoperative adjuvant after spine surgery.

With the advent of intensity-modulated radiotherapy techniques (IMRTs), anatomically precise, ablative doses of radiation can be delivered while sparing nearby critical structures, such as the spinal cord, skin, bowel, kidney, and esophagus. With advances in radiation delivery technology, less dose is delivered to these nearby organs at risk, hence minimizing the historical complications of radiation therapy. With CRT therapy treatments to the spine, the radiation is often delivered in fractions, typically 30 Gy in 10 fractions. This is done in part to minimize the toxicity of surrounding tissues and to limit the cumulative dose to the spinal cord. This technique, however, limits the radiobiological dose delivered to the intended spinal target, thereby affecting the local tumor control and the probability of progression after treatment. With SSRS, higher radiation doses are delivered to the intended targets while sparing the organs at risk. As such, SSRS has become a powerful ablative strategy with which to treat spinal metastases to maximize local tumor control.[23,24]

With fractionated CRT, external beam radiation is delivered to the target volume to minimize radiation dose to normal tissues, as discussed previously. Although this modality has demonstrated a palliative effect, the durability of local tumor control is limited by compromising on the target radiation dose due to fear of spinal cord toxicity. As a result, lower maximum radiation doses are delivered to the target volume in cases of spinal metastases, leading to a lower local control rate for more radioresistant tumor types.[25–27] Typical radiation courses range from 30 Gy to 40 Gy in 10 Gy to 20 fractions.[27] Overall, multifraction regimens demonstrate a stabilizing effect 3 months and

6 months post-treatment, albeit at low control rates (24%–34%).[27]

In order to maximize radiation delivery to the target volume while sparing nearby sensitive structures, IMRT was developed.[28] IMRT has been shown to offer excellent protection of normal tissues including the spinal cord. The physical principles behind IMRT are an extension of the general (surgically rooted) principles underlying radiosurgery.[29] Namely, when the Gamma Knife (Elekta AB, Stockholm, Sweden) was first conceptualized by Leksell[30] for treatment of cranial lesions, the use of many small ablative doses of radiation generated by the superposition of noncoplanar 60-Co–derived gamma radiation beams attained anatomic precision through use of a stereotactic frame and registration. This strategy was built on by using linear accelerators. Linear accelerators can modulate the power of electron-based radiation, typically from a tungsten source. When used in combination with stereotactic cones it is possible to achieve high-power spherical dose distributions similar to those produced with the Gamma Knife, allowing for ablative treatment of irregular targets.

With the development of micro-multileaf collimators (mMLCs), radiation could be even more finely shaped, leading to the concept of IMRT. mMLCs make fast microadjustments in thin tungsten leaflets through which a radiation beam passes, shaping the beam to the precise shape of the target volume. By breaking each beam down into individually shaped beamlets and then reintegrating into a final shape, radiation can be delivered with sharp gradients with a single isocenter.[31]

These techniques have been harnessed to create SSRS, which allows for precise delivery of conformal, image-guided radiation with doses exceeding those conventionally delivered over a fractionated course. SSRS treatments are often delivered in 1 fraction to 3 fractions with doses up to 24 Gy in a single fraction.[32–35] The local control benefit with this modality has allowed for the development of less aggressive open surgical approaches, where there is less reliance on the surgery to remove tumor. Whereas prior surgical strategies focused on gross total resection, now many implement a separation surgery strategy, with a primary goal of decompressing the spinal cord and leaving a radiation-targetable tumor volume separated by a safe distance from the spinal cord and other vital structures.[36] Typical SSRS courses involve 18 Gy to 24 Gy delivered in a single or 2 fractions.[37] Dosing regimens for 27 Gy to 40 Gy in 3 fractions to 5 fractions also have been described.[34,38]

Current treatment paradigms are not yet standardized and often are dependent on the center, provider, specifics of anatomy, cancer type, and other factors; different types of radiation in combination with surgery will be offered to treat spinal metastases. For noncompressive lesions, CRT often is offered as a first-line treatment modality. As emphasized previously, because of the need to protect vital structures from toxic radiation dosing, for many types of tumors, CRT is not capable of delivering ablative doses in single fractions; hence, recurrence rates vary greatly by tumor type.[39]

Building on the concept that every tumor is radiosensitive if a high enough dose of radiation is given, Yamada and colleagues[35] showed the efficacy of SSRS in achieving local control was largely dependent on radiation dosing to tumor volume. Furthermore, the effect of SSRS in achieving local control was seen to be independent of tumor histology, again emphasizing the power of SSRS as a noninvasive ablative tool for achieving local control in cases of spinal metastases.[35]

The overall local control rate at 1 year varies by specific SSRS protocol used but generally speaking is as high as 80% to 90%.[25,28] Currently, work is under way to determine optimal dosing and fractionation regimens in the context of various tumor types and other potentially modulating variables. Another emerging consideration is the concept of synergy of targeted therapies with radiation therapy. A recent example of synergy has been the concurrent administration of tyrosine kinase inhibitor–vascular endothelial growth factor receptor agents with SSRS.[40,41] By targeting the pathway of cytotoxicity thought to be exploited by SSRS, axitinib has been shown to lower the risk of SSRS failure compared with radiation alone.[40] The abscopal effect, a systemic response after local SSRS in those receiving concurrent checkpoint therapy, has been reported to reduce or eliminate systemic disease.[42] Whether certain careful dosing or timing of radiotherapy can take advantage of these synergistic effects has yet to be determined but serves as another potential avenue that can maximize minimally invasive ablative strategies. Prospective randomized comparisons of CRT and SSRS are currently under way (Canadian Cancer Trials, NCT02512965, comparing spine SSRS of 25 Gy in 2 fractions with CRT of 20 Gy in 5 fractions) and will be important in developing data-driven protocols to approach treatment of spinal metastases.

Although SSRS achieves higher local control,[43] it takes longer to plan and implement than CRT. In cases of radiation needed quickly due to symptomatic compression that cannot be treated with surgery, CRT may be a more appropriate treatment option.[44] In general, when planning a course of radiation, technical capability, patient tolerance and preference, goals of care, oncologic type, and surgical candidacy must all be considered in a multidisciplinary fashion, with the final plan created on an individual basis.

As radiotherapy techniques evolve, there likely will be further refinement in the ability to deliver high doses of radiation to precisely, image-defined tumor volumes. When these strategies are combined with brachytherapy as well as other ablative techniques, further improvement in durable local control hopefully can be looked forward to. Just as there has been a paradigm shift in ability to achieve local control since the advent of SSRS, there will be a paradigm shift following the ability to obtain separation and cytoreduction with minimal morbidity that comes with the optimization of minimally invasive ablative strategies.

SUMMARY

With the exception of SSRS, currently evolving ablative techniques, such as LITT, RFA, and cryoablation, are backed by only limited experience and data. Advancing optimal outcomes for the patient with metastatic cancer relies on achieving local control, managing symptoms, and tailoring the treatment approach to an individual patient's goals of care.

REFERENCES

1. Tatsui CE, Stafford RJ, Li J, et al. Utilization of laser interstitial thermotherapy guided by real-time thermal MRI as an alternative to separation surgery in the management of spinal metastasis. J Neurosurg Spine 2015;23(4):400–11.

2. Tatsui CE, Nascimento CNG, Suki D, et al. Image guidance based on MRI for spinal interstitial laser thermotherapy: technical aspects and accuracy. J Neurosurg Spine 2017;26(5):605–12.

3. Moussazadeh N, Evans LT, Grasu R, et al. Laser interstitial thermal therapy of the spine: technical aspects. Neurosurg Focus 2018;44(VideoSuppl2):V3.

4. Thomas JG, Al-Holou WN, de Almeida Bastos DC, et al. A novel use of the intraoperative MRI for metastatic spine tumors: laser interstitial thermal therapy for percutaneous treatment of epidural metastatic spine disease. Neurosurg Clin N Am 2017;28(4):513–24.

5. Tatsui CE, Lee SH, Amini B, et al. Spinal laser interstitial thermal therapy: a novel alternative to surgery for metastatic epidural spinal cord compression. Neurosurgery 2016;79(Suppl 1):S73–82.

6. Tomasian A, Gangi A, Wallace AN, et al. Percutaneous thermal ablation of spinal metastases: recent advances and review. AJR Am J Roentgenol 2018; 210(1):142–52.

7. Halpin RJ, Bendok BR, Liu JC. Minimally invasive treatments for spinal metastases: vertebroplasty, kyphoplasty, and radiofrequency ablation. J Support Oncol 2004;2(4):339–51 [discussion: 352–5].

8. Anchala PR, Irving WD, Hillen TJ, et al. Treatment of metastatic spinal lesions with a navigational bipolar radiofrequency ablation device: a multicenter retrospective study. Pain Physician 2014;17(4): 317–27.

9. Gronemeyer DH, Schirp S, Gevargez A. Image-guided radiofrequency ablation of spinal tumors: preliminary experience with an expandable array electrode. Cancer J 2002;8(1):33–9.

10. Kam NM, Maingard J, Kok HK, et al. Combined vertebral augmentation and radiofrequency ablation in the management of spinal metastases: an update. Curr Treat Options Oncol 2017;18(12):74.

11. Wallace AN, Tomasian A, Vaswani D, et al. Radiographic local control of spinal metastases with percutaneous radiofrequency ablation and vertebral augmentation. AJNR Am J Neuroradiol 2016;37(4): 759–65.

12. Reyes M, Georgy M, Brook L, et al. Multicenter clinical and imaging evaluation of targeted radiofrequency ablation (t-RFA) and cement augmentation of neoplastic vertebral lesions. J Neurointerv Surg 2018;10(2):176–82.

13. Lane MD, Le HB, Lee S, et al. Combination radiofrequency ablation and cementoplasty for palliative treatment of painful neoplastic bone metastasis: experience with 53 treated lesions in 36 patients. Skeletal Radiol 2011;40(1):25–32.

14. Madaelil TP, Wallace AN, Jennings JW. Radiofrequency ablation alone or in combination with cementoplasty for local control and pain palliation of sacral metastases: preliminary results in 11 patients. Skeletal Radiol 2016;45(9):1213–9.

15. Munk PL, Rashid F, Heran MK, et al. Combined cementoplasty and radiofrequency ablation in the treatment of painful neoplastic lesions of bone. J Vasc Interv Radiol 2009;20(7):903–11.

16. Tomasian A, Wallace A, Northrup B, et al. Spine cryoablation: pain palliation and local tumor control for vertebral metastases. AJNR Am J Neuroradiol 2016;37(1):189–95.

17. Gage AA, Baust JG. Cryosurgery for tumors - a clinical overview. Technology Cancer Res Treat 2004; 3(2):187–99.

18. Gage AA, Baust JG. Cryosurgery for tumors. J Am Coll Surg 2007;205(2):342–56.

19. Rybak LD. Fire and ice: thermal ablation of musculoskeletal tumors. Radiol Clin North Am 2009;47(3): 455–69.

20. Callstrom MR, Dupuy DE, Solomon SB, et al. Percutaneous image-guided cryoablation of painful metastases involving bone: multicenter trial. Cancer 2013;119(5):1033–41.

21. Saliken JC, McKinnon JG, Gray R. CT for monitoring cryotherapy. AJR Am J Roentgenol 1996;166(4): 853–5.

22. Campbell SC, Krishnamurthi V, Chow G, et al. Renal cryosurgery: experimental evaluation of treatment parameters. Urology 1998;52(1):29–33 [discussion: 33–4].

23. Al-Omair A, Masucci L, Masson-Cote L, et al. Surgical resection of epidural disease improves local control following postoperative spine stereotactic body radiotherapy. Neuro Oncol 2013;15(10): 1413–9.

24. Patchell RA, Tibbs PA, Regine WF, et al. Direct decompressive surgical resection in the treatment of spinal cord compression caused by metastatic cancer: a randomised trial. Lancet 2005;366(9486): 643–8.

25. Alghamdi M, Tseng CL, Myrehaug S, et al. Postoperative stereotactic body radiotherapy for spinal metastases. Chin Clin Oncol 2017;6(Suppl 2):S18.

26. Bilsky MH, Laufer I, Burch S. Shifting paradigms in the treatment of metastatic spine disease. Spine (Phila Pa 1976) 2009;34(22 Suppl):S101–7.

27. Sprave T, Hees K, Bruckner T, et al. The influence of fractionated radiotherapy on the stability of spinal bone metastases: a retrospective analysis from 1047 cases. Radiat Oncol 2018;13(1):134.

28. Tao R, Bishop AJ, Brownlee Z, et al. Stereotactic body radiation therapy for spinal metastases in the postoperative setting: a secondary analysis of mature phase 1-2 trials. Int J Radiat Oncol Biol Phys 2016;95(5):1405–13.

29. Heron DE, Gerszten K, Selvaraj RN, et al. Conventional 3D conformal versus intensity-modulated radiotherapy for the adjuvant treatment of gynecologic malignancies: a comparative dosimetric study of dose-volume histograms. Gynecol Oncol 2003; 91(1):39–45.

30. Leksell L. The stereotaxic method and radiosurgery of the brain. Acta Chir Scand 1951;102(4):316–9.

31. Agazaryan N, Solberg TD. Segmental and dynamic intensity-modulated radiotherapy delivery techniques for micro-multileaf collimator. Med Phys 2003;30(7):1758–67.

32. Laufer I, Bilsky MH. Advances in the treatment of metastatic spine tumors: the future is not what it used to be. J Neurosurg Spine 2019;30(3):299–307.

33. Tseng CL, Soliman H, Myrehaug S, et al. Imaging-based outcomes for 24 Gy in 2 daily fractions for patients with de novo spinal metastases treated with spine stereotactic body radiation therapy (SBRT). Int J Radiat Oncol Biol Phys 2018;102(3):499–507.

34. Sahgal A, Larson DA, Chang EL. Stereotactic body radiosurgery for spinal metastases: a critical review. Int J Radiat Oncol Biol Phys 2008;71(3):652–65.

35. Yamada Y, Katsoulakis E, Laufer I, et al. The impact of histology and delivered dose on local control of spinal metastases treated with stereotactic radiosurgery. Neurosurg Focus 2017;42(1):E6.

36. Moulding HD, Elder JB, Lis E, et al. Local disease control after decompressive surgery and adjuvant high-dose single-fraction radiosurgery for spine metastases. J Neurosurg Spine 2010;13(1):87–93.

37. Redmond KJ, Lo SS, Soltys SG, et al. Consensus guidelines for postoperative stereotactic body radiation therapy for spinal metastases: results of an international survey. J Neurosurg Spine 2017;26(3): 299–306.

38. Zeng KL, Tseng CL, Soliman H, et al. Stereotactic body radiotherapy (SBRT) for oligometastatic spine metastases: an overview. Front Oncol 2019;9:337.

39. Katagiri H, Takahashi M, Inagaki J, et al. Clinical results of nonsurgical treatment for spinal metastases. Int J Radiat Oncol Biol Phys 1998;42(5):1127–32.

40. Miller JA, Balagamwala EH, Angelov L, et al. Spine stereotactic radiosurgery with concurrent tyrosine kinase inhibitors for metastatic renal cell carcinoma. J Neurosurg Spine 2016;25(6):766–74.

41. Rao SS, Thompson C, Cheng J, et al. Axitinib sensitization of high Single Dose Radiotherapy. Radiother Oncol 2014;111(1):88–93.

42. Postow MA, Callahan MK, Barker CA, et al. Immunologic correlates of the abscopal effect in a patient with melanoma. N Engl J Med 2012;366(10):925–31.

43. Chang UK, Cho WI, Kim MS, et al. Local tumor control after retreatment of spinal metastasis using stereotactic body radiotherapy; comparison with initial treatment group. Acta Oncol 2012;51(5):589–95.

44. Lee JH, Lee SH. Selecting the appropriate radiation therapy technique for malignant spinal cord compression syndrome. Front Oncol 2019;9:65.

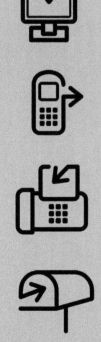

 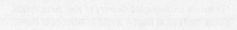

Printed and bound by CPI Group (UK) Ltd, Croydon, CR0 4YY

08/05/2025

01864747-0013